SOMERSIZE
CHOCOLATE

ALSO BY SUZANNE SOMERS

Touch Me

Keeping Secrets

Wednesday's Children

Suzanne Somers' Eat Great, Lose Weight

Suzanne Somers' Get Skinny on Fabulous Food

After the Fall

365 Ways to Change Your Life

Suzanne Somers' Eat, Cheat, and Melt the Fat Away

Somersize Desserts

Suzanne Somers' Fast and Easy

The Sexy Years

SOMERSIZE

CHOCOLATE

SUZANNE SOMERS

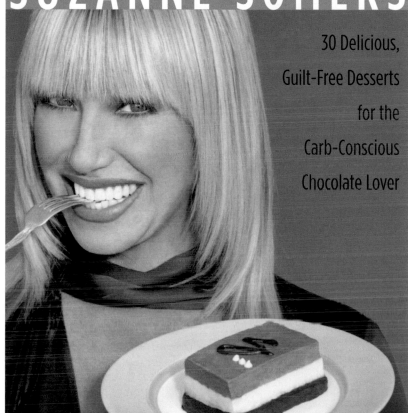

30 Delicious,

Guilt-Free Desserts

for the

Carb-Conscious

Chocolate Lover

CROWN PUBLISHERS,

Published by Crown Publishers, New York, New York.
Member of the Crown Publishing Group, a division of Random House, Inc.
www.crownpublishing.com

CROWN is a trademark and the Crown colophon is a registered trademark of Random House, Inc.

Printed in the United States of America

Design by Lauren Dong

Library of Congress Cataloging-in-Publication Data
Somers, Suzanne
        Somersize chocolate: 30 delicious, guilt-free desserts for the carb-conscious chocolate lover /
Suzanne Somers.—1st ed.
                              p.   cm.
            1. Sugar-free diet—Recipes.   2. Cookery (Chocolate)   I. Title.
RM237.85.S658   2004
641.5'63837—dc22   2003028310

ISBN 1-4000-5329-3

10 9 8 7 6 5 4 3 2 1

First Edition

To all those who share the glorious affliction of being a chocolate lover…
this one's for you!

Contents

Acknowledgments

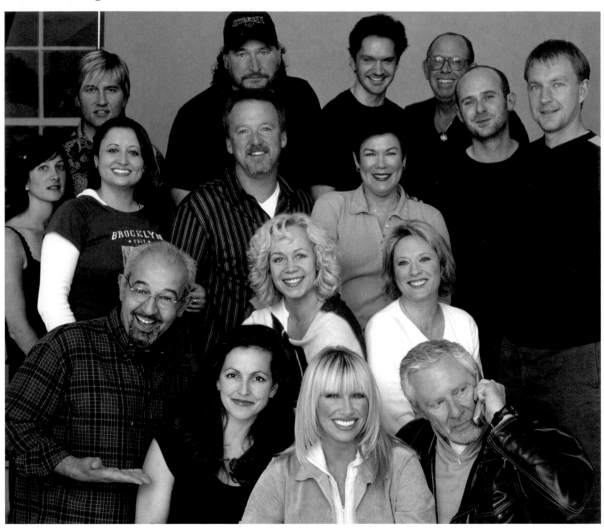

This is my sixth book in the Somersize series, and my core team remains steadfast and true. It begins with my daughter-in-law, Caroline Somers, who has been with me from the start. She was sent to me as a present all those years ago when my son Bruce chose her as his wife. She is smart, talented, and has the greatest "palate" of anyone I know. She adds the "Italian" twist in the Somersize foods, and that is why our food and recipes burst with great flavor. Thanks, Caroline, you are key to this success.

Denise Vivaldo is the head of my test kitchen and food styling team. Her bright red lips are as vibrant as her sparkling personality. Thanks to you and your awesome team: Andy Sheen-Turner, Cindie Flannigan, and Kelly Kilgo. You make me look good, and you make it taste great!

To my wonderful photographer, Jeff Katz, and his team of Jack Coyier, Victor Boghossian, Andy Strauss, and Stuart Gow. You are not only the best at what you do, you are a joy to be around. These photos make me want to lick the pages of this book! You've done it again.

To Brian Toffoli, my tabletop stylist, who makes it all look effortless. You have a wonderful ability to combine my own collection with just the right accessories. I love the look you have created. Many thanks to your assistant, Suzanne Neiderhoff.

To the beauty squad, starting with the fabulous Mooney on hair. It is such a pleasure to have you in my life . . . and to have your comb in my hair!

And thanks to Andrea Wolf for helping with my wardrobe.

To Sarah D'Agostino, you have become an integral part of the Somersize team. Thanks for organizing the shoot and helping facilitate every step of this book. To Marsha Yanchuck, for all that you do, including invaluable editing. To Anka Brazzell for keeping me scheduled, and to Liz Kozakowski, my assistant extraordinaire.

To my awesome editor, Kristin Kiser. We've become quite the team! There's no one else I would rather work with.

For the support of all my friends at Crown, headed by Jenny Frost with Steve Ross, Philip Patrick, Tina Constable, and Tammy Blake.

A big thanks to my production team at Crown, including Amy Boorstein, Jean Lynch, Linnea Knollmueller, and Lauren Dong. Thanks to Mary Schuck and Dan Rembert for another great cover design, and to Ellen Rubinstein for pulling it all together.

And to Marc Chamlin, my attorney who has bridged all the legal and business issues so effortlessly and who really cares.

Lastly, a huge thanks to Al Lowman, my literary agent and dear friend.

And to my favorite recipe tester and the best partner a girl could ask for, Alan Hamel.

My sincere thanks to all of you. I couldn't do it without you!

Back row (from left to right): Mooney, Jeff Katz, Andy Sheen-Turner, Andrew Strauss, Stuart Gow, Jack Coyier. Third row (from left to right):Andrea Wolf, Sarah D'Agostino, Brian Toffoil, Denise Vivaldo. Second row (from left to right): Victor Boghossian, Suzanne Neiderhoff, Cindie Flannigan. First row (from left to right): Caroline Somers, Suzanne Somers, Alan Hamel

Introduction

Chocolate. Mmmmmmm. Just the sound of the word makes you swoon. Chocolate: that magical, mystical, creamy creation. Chocolate: the ultimate pleasure. Chocolate: the rich, sinful temptation. When the craving hits, there's no denying it. It's the supreme "feel good" food, the sensuous gift that says, "I love you" or "I'm sorry" or "Will you marry me?" Chocolate says it all. It's sex in a foil wrapper. . . . In fact, to those of us who are absolutely nuts for the stuff, sometimes it's even better than sex!

True chocolate lovers understand the addiction. I am a person who physically needs chocolate. I need it daily and I eat it daily. I especially need it on certain days of the month. Chocolate lovers around the world understand the addiction because we speak the same language—a language of love for chocolate. Chocolate is part of a worldwide culture. Remember the film Chocolat? Or Like Water for Chocolate? Both films were about passion and how chocolate can spark that passion. For those of us who are afflicted, we are drawn to it and nothing can keep us away.

What is it that fuels our passion for chocolate? Chocolate acts as our friend, our mother, and our lover all in one. It's something we go to when we're a little down or when we get a boo-boo or when we need some affection. I'm not saying we should, but we do! When that creamy, dreamy sensation hits your tongue, the world suddenly seems an easier place to be in.

As with most sinful pleasures, overconsumption of chocolate can bring negative effects, namely, guilt. We feel guilty about the sugar, the fat, the calories, and the carbohydrates. Well, frankly, I'm too old and too wise for guilt (I had enough of it in Catholic school!). So I've found a way around the guilt. First of all, I've gotta have my chocolate. There is no getting around that. Second, I have to be able to keep my good health. And third, I need to keep my waistline from expanding. The answer? Somersize Chocolate. The key is that all the desserts in this book are made with SomerSweet Chocolate. That means you get the goodness of smooth, creamy chocolate without any of the refined sugars. As for the fat, calories, and carbohydrates, SomerSweet Chocolate falls into my Somersize weight-loss plan as an acceptable treat. It's lower in carbohydrates because we've eliminated the major source of carbs, the refined sugar! As for the fat and calories, we don't count fat grams or calories when we Somersize. In fact, we don't count anything . . . just our blessings as we drop the unwanted pounds even while indulging in decadent foods, especially chocolate!

The best news of all is that recent medical studies have shown that consuming chocolate can actually help increase our health, especially with regard to heart health. Studies done by the Mayo Clinic, the University of California, and Pennsylvania State University report that chocolate contains phytonutrients, which have been linked to the prevention of cancer and heart disease. Phytonutrients are also found in fruits, vegetables, coffee, and green tea. A Harvard study showed that men who ate chocolate lived about one year longer than men who did not. And you know they led happier lives since they were eating chocolate!

Chocolate also contains antioxidants or flavonoids, which have been shown to prevent cardiovascular disease. Antioxidants fight free radicals and can prevent damage to tissues and cells. If you're a dark chocolate lover, this is especially good news for you, since dark chocolate has about two times as many antioxidants as milk chocolate.

For those of you counting calories, chocolate is high in calories but not in cholesterol. The Mayo Clinic study showed that flavonoids help raise good cholesterol and lower bad cholesterol. The moral of the story: add some dark chocolate to your diet! It not only tastes great, but it may also actually help you stay healthier!

I'll take my chocolate fix in just about any form. I love a great chocolate truffle in the afternoon or a piece of a chocolate bar. As for dessert, my first choice is chocolate cake. Of course, I'll take a decadent chocolate soufflé any day of the week, and I am crazy about chocolate ice cream and rich, creamy chocolate pudding. Let's not forget brownies, fudge, tarts, cheesecake, mousse, petit fours, and more!

In this book you'll see my passion for chocolate. I have developed more than thirty mouthwatering desserts using milk chocolate, dark chocolate, white chocolate, or some combination of the three. Many of these desserts are simple to make, but others are more labor-intensive for those more advanced in the culinary arts. The advanced recipes are not necessarily difficult; they just take more time. Either way, make sure to follow the directions exactly. It makes my heart sink when I get a letter or an e-mail saying that a recipe failed. Often it is because the ingredients weren't measured accurately or because substitutions were made. Baking is a science and a wonderful experiment in chemistry. Since these desserts are made without refined sugars, they have been tested very carefully to make sure they work. Even with careful testing, there can be variations in baking based upon altitude, humidity, and differing heat in ovens. Read the following sections for tips that can help you get perfect results.

Of all the cookbooks I have written, none has been more fun than this one. What could be better than a complete book about chocolate? Testing these wonderful recipes has been heavenly! And unlike cooking with refined sugar and chocolate, I have had the added benefit of keeping my weight in control. With Somersize Chocolate you can have your chocolate cake and eat it, too!

CHOCOLATE HISTORY

How in the world did someone ever figure out that the pod of the cacao tree could create the most legendary and romantic desserts of all time? The Spaniards usually get the credit, but the actual cacao tree is said to have originated in South America, where the Aztecs and Mayans discovered it. In A.D. 600 the Mayans established the earliest known cocoa plantations. The Mayans and Aztecs took pods from the cacao tree and made a drink they called xocoatl. Aztec legend has it that cacao seeds were brought from Paradise; anyone who ate the fruit of the cacao tree gained wisdom and power. I still believe that! No wonder I love my chocolate.

Christopher Columbus brought cacao beans to King Ferdinand after his fourth visit to the New World, but the sensation didn't catch on. It wasn't until 1519 that Spanish explorer Hernando Cortés discovered the power of chocolate when he visited Emperor Montezuma of Mexico. Cortés noticed that the emperor's beverage of choice was chocolatl, a mixture of chocolate, vanilla, and spices mixed to a thick frothy consistency and served cold. Montezuma drank chocolatl before entering his harem, which led to the belief that it was a powerful aphrodisiac. Hey, whatever works!

Cortés took chocolate back to Spain, where

monks kept chocolate processing a secret for nearly a century. It was a profitable industry for Spain, which planted cacao trees in its overseas colonies. However, with the decline of Spain's power, the secret of cacao leaked out at last, and the Spanish Crown's monopoly over chocolate came to an end. Knowledge of it soon spread throughout France, Italy, Germany, and England.

The first shop to actually sell chocolate opened in London in 1657. Chocolate was so pricey that it was considered a beverage only for the elite class. It was also used as a medicinal remedy by physicians of the day who would prescribe it for various maladies. It still cures most of my ills!

The first chocolate factory in the United States was established in Dorchester, Massachusetts, in 1765. Chocolate was made from cocoa beans imported from the West Indies.

In 1828 Conrad Van Houten of the Netherlands developed a way of mechanically extracting the fat (cacao butter) from cacao liquor. The leftover solids could then be ground into cocoa powder. Confectioners now had the two ingredients they needed to make solid chocolate: cocoa butter and cocoa powder. Chocolate was now on its way to becoming an inexpensive treat, rather than a luxury for the rich.

In 1897 Rodolphe Lindt from Switzerland developed a process of grinding roasted cacao to smooth out the inherent grittiness. This process, known as conching, sometimes took as long as two or three days, but it gave chocolate a silky texture and a smooth melt. Chocolate could now be made cheaply and on a huge scale. Everyone could afford it, and the chocolate craze began!

The first chocolate bars were made from bittersweet chocolate. What we know as milk chocolate did not originate until 1875, when Henri Nestlé, a Swiss manufacturer of condensed milk, and Daniel Peter, a chocolate maker, got together and decided to combine their products. Today milk chocolate is the most popular type of chocolate in the world.

The 1893 World's Columbian Exposition in Chicago displayed German chocolate-making machinery, and Milton Hershey, a very successful maker of caramels, saw the potential for chocolate. He soon installed the machinery in his factory, and the great love affair between chocolate and caramel was born.

During World War I, the U.S. Army commissioned various American chocolate manufacturers to ship twenty- to forty-pound blocks of chocolate to army bases. The blocks were cut into smaller pieces and distributed to soldiers in Europe. Eventually, manufacturers started making smaller pieces themselves. By the time soldiers arrived home with their fondness for chocolate, the American candy bar business was in full swing. Candy bar manufacturers became established throughout the United States in the 1920s, making thousands of different types of candy bars.

Today the chocolate industry in the United States absorbs more than a quarter of the world's production of cacao. U.S. consumers spend more than 7 billion dollars a year on chocolate and eat 2.8 billion pounds of it annually (about 12 pounds per person), nearly half of the world's supply. Chocolate is currently the most popular candy being sold.

CHOCOLATE PRODUCTION

Having been in the chocolate business for the past several years, I have become familiar with terms such as "chocolate nibs," "chocolate liquor," "cocoa powder," "cocoa butter," "bittersweet," "unsweetened," "semisweet," and many more. Now that I understand how chocolate is made, these terms are easy to categorize.

Chocolate is made from the pods of the cacao tree, which grows in South America, Africa, the West Indies, and parts of America and the Far East. Each pod is sliced open to reveal twenty-five to fifty almond-shaped seeds or beans. The seeds and surrounding pulp are allowed to ferment in the sun for two to three days. The seeds are then dried for several days or even weeks.

These dried seeds are shipped to chocolate manufacturers, where they are roasted over low heat. It is at this point that the seed begins to develop its distinctive chocolate flavor and scent. After this, the shells are removed from the seeds and the remaining kernels, or "nibs," are used for making chocolate. The next step is "conching," a grinding process where most of the cocoa butter is removed, leaving a thick paste called "chocolate liquor." Many people are confused by this term, thinking it is chocolate with alcohol. Chocolate liquor is simply unsweetened chocolate paste. This paste is then molded to form unsweetened chocolate, as we commonly know it.

Cocoa powder is made by grinding even more cocoa butter from the kernels. This drier chocolate paste is then ground into a powder resulting in cocoa powder.

TYPES OF CHOCOLATE

Just as there are connoisseurs of fine wine and coffee, there are also those with a discerning palate for chocolate. What type is the best? From what region? How is it ground, blended, and sweetened to make the perfect bar? The answer is in our taste buds! We all have our favorites—from the inexpensive drugstore candy bar to the finest Belgian truffle, the judgment of the best chocolate is as unique as we are. Here are the various types of chocolate.

Unsweetened Chocolate

Unsweetened chocolate contains no sugar and is used in recipes containing other sweet ingredients. As I mentioned earlier, unsweetened chocolate can also be called chocolate liquor or chocolate nibs. Grocery stores carry unsweetened baking chocolate that usually comes in squares or chips. Common brands are Hershey's and Baker's. For higher-quality brands, look for Valrhona, Ghirardelli, and Scharffen Berger in fine candy stores or gourmet food markets.

Semisweet, Bittersweet, and Extra-Bittersweet Dark Chocolate

When the chocolate liquor is combined with sugar and extra cocoa butter, it becomes sweetened chocolate. Semisweet, bittersweet, and extra-bittersweet chocolate are all terms for sweetened chocolate. Semisweet is the sweetest of the three, then bittersweet, then extra-bittersweet, although the level of sweetness varies from manufacturer to manufacturer. All of these chocolates are used in baking and can be interchanged as long as you adjust for the sweetness by adding or taking away additional sugar or sweetener in the recipe. A dip of your finger into the batter will tell you whether you want to adjust the sweetness level.

All of these sweetened chocolates are dark chocolate, the type most commonly used in cooking. One of the ways to determine the quality of your dark chocolate is by the amount of cocoa solids. Dark chocolate contains anywhere from 30 percent to 75 percent cocoa solids. In general, the higher the cocoa content the higher the quality. In my first few Somersize books I did not yet have SomerSweet and I always recommended using dark chocolate with at least 60 percent cocoa. This ensures that you are getting more cocoa and less fillers, including sugars! The higher the percentage of cocoa, the less sweet and more intense the chocolate becomes. When I was using this low-sugar chocolate for cooking, I went all the way up to 75 percent cocoa solids for a rich, intense flavor. The only time you see percentages on chocolate is when you are purchasing fine chocolate. Brands such as Valrhona, Ghirardelli, and Scharffen Berger are excellent and usually provide these percentages for you.

Milk Chocolate

Milk chocolate contains milk solids, which makes for a creamy and mild flavor. Milk chocolate is sweeter than dark chocolate and is most commonly used as a snacking chocolate. It is more sensitive to heat and melts at a lower temperature than dark chocolate. Inexpensive milk chocolates can have added oils and fillers to reduce the cost. More expensive brands do not add the fillers. Milk chocolate is the most popular of all the chocolates and is the type most commonly consumed.

Although milk chocolate has a wonderful flavor and texture, as a general rule you should not substitute milk chocolate when a recipe calls for dark chocolate. If a recipe calls for semisweet chocolate, you should use dark chocolate, not milk chocolate. Remember, there are several types of dark chocolate with varying levels of sweetness. These dark chocolates are the more traditional types used in classic baking of chocolate desserts.

White Chocolate

Now for my great love . . . white chocolate! Many will say that white chocolate isn't even really considered chocolate. Call it whatever you want, I think it's divine! White chocolate does not contain cocoa solids at all, only cocoa butter. It has a higher intensity of sugar to make up for the missing cocoa (which is probably why I love it so much). Cheap brands of white chocolate are made without real cocoa butter, using oils instead. I always look for the cocoa butter on the label to make sure I'm getting better quality. White chocolate can be tricky to work with, and you should take care not to overheat it when melting. It's especially difficult to work with if you are using white chocolate made with oils instead of real cocoa butter. The oils tend to separate when melted. I have used SomerSweet White Chocolate Baking Bars in several of the desserts in this book. It has no refined sugar at all and is great for adding dramatic decorations on milk and dark chocolate desserts.

Confectionery Chocolate

Every now and then I see a recipe that calls for confectionery chocolate, also known as coating chocolate or "couverture." This is a very high-quality chocolate with the highest cocoa butter content. It is available in bittersweet, semisweet, white, and milk chocolate. Couverture is ideal for dipping because, when melted, it is very fluid. Commercial bakers use it for dipping cookies or pretzels, or for making candy. Again, cheaper types are made with oils and fillers. If you choose to seek out this type of chocolate, look for pure ingredients like cocoa solids (chocolate liquor), cocoa butter, and milk solids.

This product is not readily available, as it is usually sold on a commercial level. You may substitute regular chocolate in its place.

Cocoa Powder

Cocoa powder is the powder left after the cocoa butter has been completely pressed out of the cacao pods. It is unsweetened and has a bitter flavor. It is excellent for adding a strong chocolate flavor to recipes. Dutch-process cocoa is cocoa processed with alkali. This process makes the cocoa powder less bitter and slightly darker in color than regular cocoa powder. Cocoa powder is available at most grocery stores.

Sugar-free and No Sugar Added Chocolate

With the popularity of low-carbohydrate lifestyles and weight-loss programs, many are turning to chocolates made without refined sugars. This is how we can still have our chocolate while we are losing weight. Most chocolates of this type are made with maltitol, a sweetener that also adds creaminess. The addition of maltitol rounds out the grittiness of unsweetened chocolate; however, overconsumption of maltitol can cause a laxative effect.

When I first developed my sweetener, Somer-Sweet, I would make desserts using unsweetened chocolate and SomerSweet. The taste was good, but it did not address the grittiness of the unsweetened chocolate. Then I developed SomerSweet Chocolate Baking Bars. In fact, this entire book is designed around these bars, making these Somersize desserts guilt-free for those on my Somersize weight-loss program or any program on which you are asked to watch your carbohydrate intake.

SomerSweet Baking Bars are made with high-quality Belgian chocolate that is then sweetened with a combination of SomerSweet and maltitol. The result is simply the finest-tasting chocolate bar with absolutely no refined sugars! I took my time developing these bars, and I am proud of the result. I do not miss sugared chocolate with these bars on hand. They completely satisfy my craving without the ill effects of refined sugar.

As with regular chocolate, there are less expensive brands of sugar-free chocolate available on the market. Personally, I feel that the money is worth it to buy SomerSweet chocolate. I am not a fan of cheap chocolate, and it does not hold up in the baking process. There's nothing more disappointing than taking the effort to make a beautiful dessert and ending up with lousy results. That being said, you may use any brand of sugar-free chocolate in place of the SomerSweet chocolate called for in the recipes; however, I cannot guarantee the results. In general, if you select a different brand, look for ones that list real chocolate (chocolate, chocolate liquor, etc.) and real cocoa butter to ensure that you get similar results.

SomerSweet Baking Bars are available in dark, milk, and white. I also have a wide variety of assorted chocolates, truffles, caramels, toffee, and more. All are made without any refined sugars. You can find them at SuzanneSomers.com, and they are delicious!

STORING CHOCOLATE

Chocolate should be stored in a cool, dry environment, away from heat or sunlight. Most baking chocolate has a shelf life of about a year. To extend the shelf life of chocolate, store in the refrigerator or freezer. Just make sure to wrap the chocolate tightly to prevent it from acquiring flavors of other foods. Sometimes the chocolate will "bloom" when it gets cold. This is the cocoa butter rising to the surface. It does not affect taste and does not mean the chocolate has gone bad.

I store my wrapped baking bars in sealed plastic bags in the freezer.

COOKING WITH CHOCOLATE

A water bath or double boiler over low heat is the best way to melt chocolate, never over direct heat. Make sure that the bottom of the pan with the chocolate does not come in contact with the simmering water. Chocolate should be broken into small pieces and stirred when it begins to melt, making sure that no steam or drops of water get into the chocolate.

Chocolate can also be melted in a microwave. Break chocolate into small pieces and place in a microwave-safe bowl. Timing will vary, depending upon differences in microwaves and in quantity and type of chocolate. As a rough guide, melt 4 ounces of semisweet chocolate on high for 1 minute. Stir the chocolate, let stand for 30 seconds, then stir again. If necessary, heat in increments of 30 seconds, stirring in between until the chocolate is completely melted.

Milk chocolate is more sensitive than dark chocolate and extra care should be taken when melting.

Accurate Measuring

One of the most common mistakes made in baking is misusing dry measuring cups and liquid measuring cups. Dry measuring cups usually consist of a stack of cups, made from metal or plastic, that nestle inside one another. These cups should be used to measure all dry ingredients, such as flour, sugar, or sugar substitutes, and heavy, thick, wet ingredients like sour cream. Fill the ingredients over the edge of the cup, then use the flat side of a knife to scrape off the ingredients until they are level with the cup.

Liquid cups are usually made from glass or plastic with a pourable spout. They list measurements in ounces and in cups and are used to measure liquids such as water, cream, milk, and lemon juice. To accurately measure, lower your eye level to the counter to check the line of liquid in the cup rather than lifting the cup to your eye line. When lifting the cup to your eye line you can inadvertently tip the level of the liquid and get a faulty measurement.

For measuring spoons, overfill your ingredients, then scrape the excess with the flat side of a knife until they are level with the spoon.

Line Up, Read Through

This may sound like common sense, but one of the most important recipes for success in the kitchen is to line up all the ingredients on the counter before beginning any recipe. This ensures that nothing will get left out. Next, make sure to read the entire recipe before beginning. How many times have you been caught by surprise because you didn't read the whole recipe? Take the extra few moments to lay out the recipe in your head before you dive in and make mistakes.

SomerSweet

All of the recipes in this book are sweetened with SomerSweet, my answer to sugar. This wonderful product is the anchor of my entire line of Somersize food products. It is a fabulous alternative to sugar because it bakes like sugar, it tastes like sugar, and it even caramelizes! SomerSweet is five times sweeter than sugar; but unlike other sweeteners, SomerSweet holds up to heat in the baking process. Many other products become bitter when heated. SomerSweet does not have a nasty aftertaste, just the sweetness you want without any of the refined sugars.

Controlling your sugar and carbohydrate intake is the key to my Somersize weight-loss program.

Now it's even easier to stay on the program because you can have something sweet without having refined sugar. With less than one gram of carbohydrates and zero sugars per serving, it's a great choice for anyone who understands the health benefits of a low-sugar diet.

SomerSweet has been specially formulated for individuals who want to control their sugar intake and maintain normal blood sugar levels. Somer-Sweet is a delicious blend of oligofructose, inulin, fructose, sprouted mung bean extract, and acesulfame K. Oligofructose and inulin are sweet fibers derived from chicory. The bit of fructose is naturally occurring in these sweet fibers; we do not add it to the blend, and it's such a small amount that our nutrition label boasts zero sugars per serving under the FDA guidelines for labeling. Acesulfame K is a nonnutritive sweetener that is fed to a mung bean plant along with water. When the mung bean plant sprouts, the leaves become sweet with only a touch of the acesulfame K in the sweet extract that is used in the finished product. This incredible combination of ingredients adds up to a product that tastes amazing, bakes beautifully, and that you can feel good about using.

I get many questions from diabetics asking if SomerSweet is safe for them. If you are diabetic, please check with your doctor to see if SomerSweet is right for you. We have many diabetics who use the product and love it, but please put your health before your taste buds and make sure SomerSweet is approved by your doctor.

SomerSweet is available in cans, packets, or by the case at SuzanneSomers.com.

Flour

Unlike other low-carb programs, when you Somersize, you are allowed to have carbohydrates as long as they are whole-grain. That means we can use whole-wheat flour but not white flour. Recently I discovered a new type of whole-wheat flour that is made from a white kernel of wheat. It is called "white whole-wheat flour." Please do not confuse this with "white wheat flour," which is simply white flour that originated from a kernel of wheat, only to be refined down to white flour. White whole-wheat flour is the whole grain of white wheat. I highly recommend it for baking. It is ground very fine, which helps it bake like regular white flour while retaining its whole-grain goodness. In fact, all of my Somersize Bread Mixes are made with this flour, as well as my Blueberry Muffin Mix.

If you can't find white whole-wheat flour, try whole-wheat pastry flour. The pastry flour is ground more finely than regular whole-wheat flour and will give a better result in baking.

White whole-wheat flour is available at health food stores and gourmet markets. Look for King Arthur brand or go to their website at www.kingarthurflour.com. If you are not a Somersizer and want to use regular white flour, simply substitute all-purpose white flour.

Beaten Egg Whites

Many of the recipes in this book call for beaten egg whites. Especially in the absence of flour, beaten egg whites add volume to chocolate cakes, meringues, soufflés, and more. Here are some tips on how to beat the egg whites to ensure great results.

Egg whites can be beaten with an electric mixer or with a wire whisk. Either way, your bowl and beaters must be perfectly clean and dry. Even a tiny drop of water or a small amount of egg yolk can lessen your results. You need the egg white to become light and fluffy to make your dessert rise properly. Water or fat can inhibit this process.

Beat your egg whites right before you need them. The egg whites will fall if you beat them in advance. You want to beat them just before folding into the batter and then bake your dessert immediately.

Be careful not to overbeat your egg whites. Egg whites are usually beaten until soft peaks form. This means that when you lift your whisk or beater out of the egg whites, the whites will just hold their form; but they should still be soft peaks. Test frequently to ensure that you do not overbeat or the egg whites will become stiff. Stiff egg whites mean that the peaks will hold their form and look a bit dry. When overbeaten, the egg whites can even develop a slightly "curdled" look. If they become too stiff or dry, start over with a fresh batch. They will not fold into the batter if they are too stiff, and there is no sense in wasting good batter and expensive chocolate with overbeaten egg whites.

The exception to the rule is when you are making meringue. In this case you will beat your egg whites until they are quite stiff. The sugar or sweetener added will also help to stiffen the egg whites. In these recipes the stiffened egg whites become the entire batter, rather than being folded into a batter.

A copper bowl and a wire whisk are the best tools for getting airy, fluffy, perfectly beaten egg whites. Copper bowls are expensive, but they do make you feel like a real chef!

Folding Ingredients

When a recipe tells you to "fold" one ingredient into another, it is so that you keep the volume of air in the finished batter. This technique takes practice. You need to make sure you thoroughly incorporate the ingredients; but if you fold too vigorously, you will lose the air in your beaten egg whites or whipped cream and lose volume in the finished product.

Fold your ingredients together right after your egg whites or cream have been whipped to perfection. Make sure you have a large rubber spatula and a good-size bowl so that you can make large, round strokes. Generally, you fold the lighter, beaten ingredients into the heavier batter. Place the beaten egg whites or whipped cream on top of the batter. Hold the bowl in one hand, then glide the spatula down the side in the bowl, along the bottom, then up and over the beaten ingredients. This method takes the batter and gently folds it over the beaten

ingredients to retain the fluffiness. Keep turning the bowl and folding in this manner until the egg whites have thoroughly mixed with the batter. You do not want chunks of egg white floating in the batter. The end result should be a light, fluffy mixture of batter and egg whites.

Check Oven Temperature

I have two homes with two entirely different ovens. At my Los Angeles home, my oven seems to cook at just the right temperature. At my desert home, my ovens seem to run a little cooler. I am constantly adjusting the temperature to get it right. Both of these ovens are considered commercial-quality, professional ovens. At first I denied that my oven could be at fault. Now I realize that all ovens heat slightly differently, and the only way to be sure is to use an oven thermometer.

Since I have not worked in your kitchen, I highly recommend you get yourself a good oven thermometer to make sure your oven is at the correct temperature. Being off by 50 degrees can make a huge difference in your baking results.

Pastry Bags

In many recipes I use a pastry bag to insert fillings or decorate. These bags are inexpensive and can be purchased at any cooking store. They are usually canvas on the outside and plastic-lined on the inside. If you do not have a pastry bag, simply use a plastic baggie and snip off the end.

To fill the pastry bag, place it tip side down into a tall glass or jar. Fold down the top edge a few inches, then spoon in the filling. When filled, unfold the sides of the bag and twist from the top down. This will ensure that the filling does not spill out the top of the bag. Continue piping or decorating by twisting down from the top of the bag, then refill as necessary.

Making Substitutions

All of the recipes in this book have been made with SomerSweet and SomerSweet Baking Chocolate so that we can enjoy these treats without guilt! This is how they have been tested and how I feel they taste best. If you prefer to use other brands of sugar-free chocolate or other sweeteners, feel free to do so; but I cannot attest to the results. As I mentioned above, for substitutions please use the best quality chocolate you can find. As for other sweeteners, I have not had much luck baking with saccharin or aspartame, so I have not provided measurements for these products. Remember, SomerSweet is approximately five times sweeter than sugar. If you want to use sucralose (Splenda) in place of SomerSweet you will need substantially more, since sucralose is the same sweetness as sugar. To bake with sucralose, follow the same measurements for sugar.

For those who want to make these desserts with sugar and sugared chocolate, I have provided measurements for each recipe in a side box.

Happy Baking! Enjoy, Suzanne Somers

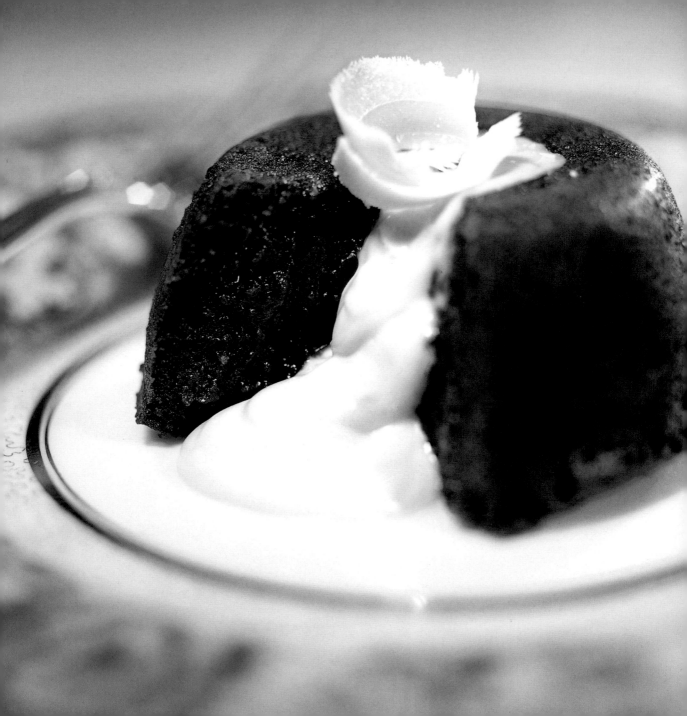

MOLTEN CHOCOLATE CAKE WITH WHITE CHOCOLATE LAVA

LEVEL TWO   Makes 6 servings

Your friends will be impressed by this one; These divine individual chocolate cakes have a gooey surprise inside—a river of white chocolate lava!

Preheat oven to 325°. Butter six small glass custard cups (6 ounces each, 4 inches wide).

In a double boiler, heat the dark chocolate and the butter, stirring until smooth. Set aside.

Place the eggs, egg yolks, and SomerSweet into a large bowl. Beat with an electric mixer until pale and thickened, about 10 minutes. Add the melted dark chocolate and the flour, then beat for 5 more minutes. Pour half the mixture into the custard cups, filling them nearly halfway. Divide the white chocolate among the custard cups, placing it in the center of the batter. Pour the rest of the batter on top. Place the cups into the oven and bake for about 12 minutes, or until the sides seem stiff but the centers jiggle when touched.

Let cups cool for a few minutes before sliding a knife around the sides of each to loosen. Invert each onto a dessert plate. Prick the centers with a fork and split open so the melted chocolate in the center oozes out. Garnish with whipped cream, raspberries, or white chocolate curls.

PERFECTLY WHIPPED CREAM
PRO/FATS—LEVEL ONE   Makes 10–12 servings

My classic whipped cream made with SomerSweet.

Whip the cream with an electric mixer until very thick. Add the vanilla and SomerSweet. Continue whipping until soft peaks form.

---

6 ounces or 1¼ SomerSweet Dark Chocolate Baking Bars (37½ squares), chopped

11 tablespoons unsalted butter

3 large eggs

3 large egg yolks

2 tablespoons SomerSweet

¼ cup 100% white whole wheat flour (or whole wheat pastry flour)

3 ounces or ⅔ (4.9-ounce) SomerSweet White Chocolate Baking Bar (18 squares), chopped

Perfectly Whipped Cream (below), fresh raspberries, or white chocolate curls (page 65), for garnish

SUGAR SUBSTITUTIONS
½ cup sugar
7 ounces dark chocolate
4 ounces white chocolate

PERFECTLY WHIPPED CREAM

2 cups heavy cream

1 teaspoon vanilla extract

2 teaspoons SomerSweet

SUGAR SUBSTITUTIONS
¼ cup sugar

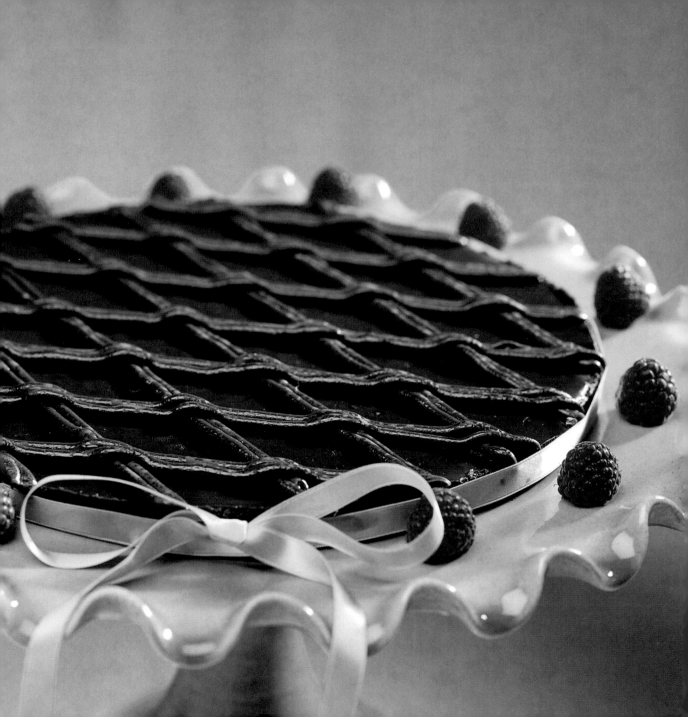

CHOCOLATE RASPBERRY TRUFFLE TART

ALMOST LEVEL ONE   Makes 8 servings

I love the look of this tart. Jam tarts are a traditional favorite . . . and they're so easy to make. You can use any of my Somersize jams for this lovely tart: strawberry, triple berry, blackberry, blueberry, or sour cherry—all taste great!

Preheat oven to 400°. Line an 8-inch springform pan with waxed or parchment paper. Grease parchment and sides of pan with butter. Set aside.

TO MAKE CRUST

Beat together the cream cheese, eggs, vanilla, SomerSweet, and cocoa powder until smooth. Pour the batter into the prepared pan. Bake for 10 minutes. Allow to cool completely.

TO MAKE FILLING

Place the unsweetened chocolate and chocolate baking bar into a small bowl. Heat the cream in a small, heavy saucepan until almost boiling and pour over the chopped chocolate. Stir until the chocolate has melted. Fold in the vanilla, SomerSweet, and butter and stir until smooth. Spread or paint a thin layer of chocolate mixture over the crust to keep the jam from soaking into the crust and making it soggy. Refrigerate until chocolate has set, about 10 minutes.

Spread the jam over the chocolate layer. Pour the remaining chocolate mixture over the jam. Refrigerate for 2 hours or overnight. Carefully run a thin-bladed knife or spatula around the edge of the pan to loosen the tart. Remove the sides of the pan. Run a metal spatula underneath the tart to loosen the waxed paper. Remove paper before serving. Decorate with melted chocolate in a lattice design, or just drizzle on top.

FOR THE CRUST
2 ounces cream cheese at
    room temperature
2 large eggs
1 teaspoon vanilla extract
1 teaspoon SomerSweet
1 tablespoon unsweetened
    cocoa powder

FOR THE FILLING
3 ounces (3 squares)
    unsweetened baking
    chocolate, chopped
1 (4.9-ounce) SomerSweet
    Dark Chocolate Baking Bar
    (30 squares), chopped
1 cup heavy cream
1 teaspoon vanilla extract
1 teaspoon SomerSweet
2 tablespoons unsalted butter
    at room temperature
1/2 cup Somersize Raspberry
    Jam

SUGAR SUBSTITUTIONS
crust: 3 tablespoons sugar
filling: 2 tablespoons sugar
        5 ounces dark chocolate

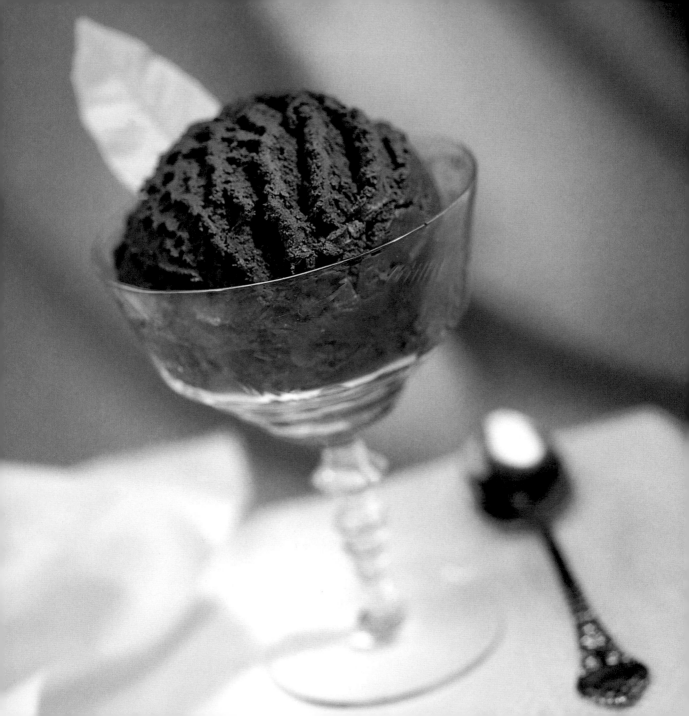

BITTERSWEET CHOCOLATE SORBET

ALMOST LEVEL ONE   Makes 4 servings

Chocolate sorbet has its own special taste . . . icy and satisfying. Sorbets are softer than sherbets and contain no milk or cream. My Bittersweet Chocolate Sorbet is a fabulous, light dessert that will melt in your mouth.

Chop the chocolate into ½-inch pieces. Place in a food processor and process until finely chopped. Set aside.

Pour the water and coffee into a small saucepan. Whisk in the SomerSweet and bring to a boil. Remove from heat. With the food processor running, slowly pour the coffee mixture through the feed tube, melting the chocolate. Continue processing until the mixture is smooth. Pour the mixture into a bowl and allow to cool to room temperature, about 20 minutes. Cover and refrigerate for 2 hours. Pour into an ice cream maker and freeze according to manufacturer's directions. Scoop into pretty dishes and garnish, as desired, with chocolate leaves.

2 (4.9-ounce) SomerSweet
   Dark Chocolate Baking Bars
   (60 squares)
1 cup water
1 cup brewed decaffeinated
   coffee
2 tablespoons SomerSweet
   Chocolate Leaves (optional;
   page 85), for garnish

SUGAR SUBSTITUTIONS
3 tablespoons sugar
10 ounces dark chocolate

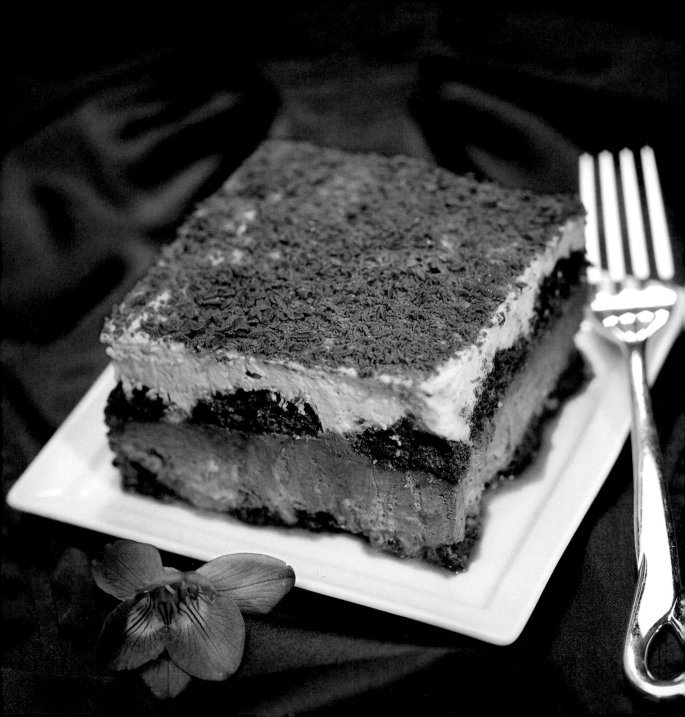

TIRAMISÙ

ALMOST LEVEL ONE   Makes 6–8 servings

To make this tiramisù, first prepare the Chocolate-Dipped Cocoa Meringue Cookies (page 81), pour the batter into a sealable bag, snip off the end, and pipe out the cookies into ladyfingers. Bake as directed, then layer the cookies with this recipe to make a great, traditional tiramisù.

TO MAKE FILLING

Beat together the mascarpone, SomerSweet, vanilla, and ¼ cup of the coffee with an electric mixer until smooth. Divide the mixture between two bowls. Add the cocoa powder to one bowl and beat until combined.

In a third bowl, beat the cream until stiff. Divide between the two bowls of mascarpone mixture. Fold in and set aside.

Place half of the cookies into an 8-inch square baking dish. Sprinkle with half of the coffee. Spoon the chocolate cheese mixture over the cookies. Sprinkle with half the grated chocolate. Layer the rest of the cookies on top of the grated chocolate and sprinkle with the remaining coffee. Spread the last of the cheese mixture over the cookies. Sprinkle with the remaining grated chocolate. Cover and refrigerate 2 hours or overnight before serving.

16 ounces mascarpone (or cream cheese), softened
1 tablespoon SomerSweet
1 teaspoon vanilla extract
1 tablespoon decaf coffee crystals dissolved in 1 cup hot water
2 tablespoons unsweetened cocoa powder
2 cups heavy cream
1 recipe Chocolate-Dipped Cocoa Meringue Cookies (page 81) (don't dip cookies into chocolate)
2.5 ounces or ½ SomerSweet Milk Chocolate Baking Bar (15 squares), grated

SUGAR SUBSTITUTIONS
¼ cup sugar
3 ounces milk chocolate

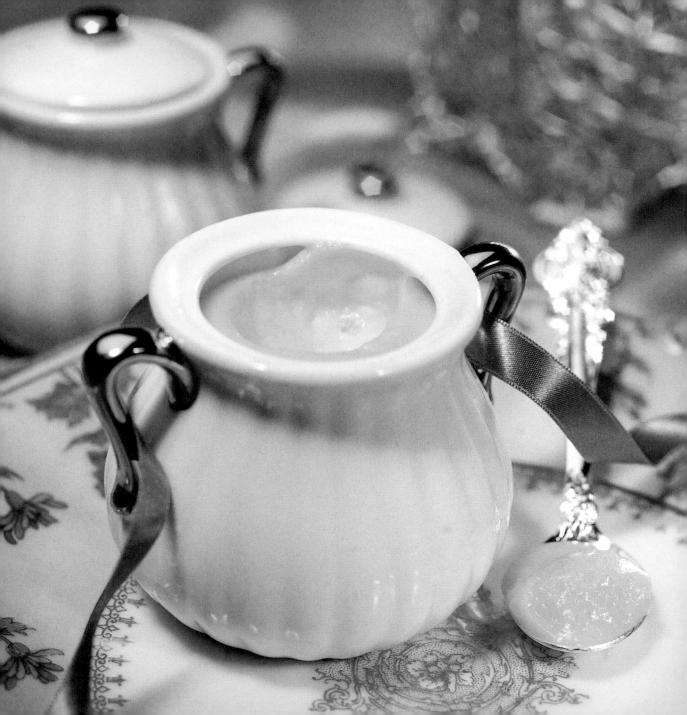

WHITE CHOCOLATE POTS DE CRÈME

ALMOST LEVEL ONE   **Makes 6 servings**

Anyone who knows me knows that I *love* white chocolate! Chocolate Pots de Crème is a fancy name for very rich French pudding. The dark chocolate version of this first appeared in *Get Skinny on Fabulous Food.* Now it's better than ever with SomerSweet chocolate, especially white chocolate! Serve it in my darling little covered pots (available on my website) for a truly authentic French dessert.

Preheat oven to 350°.

Place 1½ cups of the cream into a small, heavy saucepan over low heat. Place the remaining cream and the chocolate into the top of a double boiler over gently simmering water. Beat the yolks in a small bowl and set aside. When the cream just begins to boil, remove from the heat and stir in the SomerSweet and salt. Set aside.

Stir the chocolate mixture until perfectly smooth. Remove from the heat and gradually add the hot cream to the chocolate mixture, stirring constantly. Gradually stir the chocolate mixture into the yolks. Add the vanilla. Return the mixture to the top of a double boiler and cook over gently simmering water, stirring constantly with a rubber spatula, for 3 minutes. Pour mixture through a fine sieve or strainer into ramekins or covered pots. Don't fill all the way. Place pots into a baking dish and place baking dish into the oven. Pour very hot water into the baking dish to reach halfway up the sides of the pots. Cover the pots with lids or, if using ramekins, cover the tops of the ramekins with a baking sheet. Bake for 25 minutes. The custard will look a little soft, but will become firmer as it chills. Remove the pots from the baking dish and allow to cool. Refrigerate for 2 hours before serving. Serve with a dollop of Perfectly Whipped Cream.

2 cups heavy cream
1 (4.9-ounce) SomerSweet
   White Chocolate Baking Bar
   (30 squares), chopped
7 large egg yolks
1 tablespoon SomerSweet
Pinch salt
1 tablespoon vanilla extract
Perfectly Whipped Cream
   (page 23)

SUGAR SUBSTITUTIONS
¼ cup sugar
5 ounces white chocolate

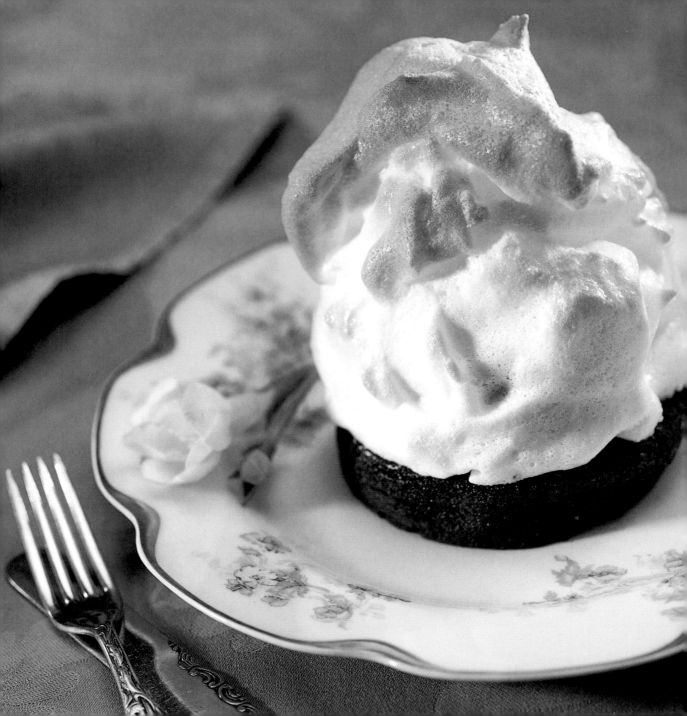

MINI COCONUT BAKED ALASKA

ALMOST LEVEL ONE   **Makes 6 servings**

This tastes awesome. You can use Somersize Coconut Ice Cream Mix and a box of Somersize Flourless Chocolate Brownie Mix to make this incredible dessert even easier. I love to make a mountain of meringue on my Baked Alaska. It looks so impressive!

TO MAKE COCONUT ICE CREAM

Pour the cream and water into a heavy saucepan. Heat until hot, but not boiling. Remove from the heat. Place the yolks into a medium bowl. Whisk for 2 minutes. Pour the cream over the eggs, whisking constantly. Pour the mixture back into the saucepan and place over low heat. Stir until the mixture thickens and coats the back of a spoon. Pour the mixture through a sieve into a clean bowl. Add the SomerSweet and coconut extract. Stir well. Cover with plastic wrap and cool to room temperature. Refrigerate for at least 2 hours. Pour into an ice cream machine and freeze according to manufacturer's directions.

TO MAKE CRUST

Preheat oven to 350°. Butter six 6-ounce ramekins and set aside.

Melt the chocolates and butter together in a double boiler over gently simmering water. Stir until the chocolate is smooth. Remove from the heat and allow mixture to cool slightly. Meanwhile, beat the eggs until pale and tripled in volume, 8 to 10 minutes (very important). Add the SomerSweet and beat for another minute. Mix one third of the egg mixture into the chocolate mixture. Carefully fold the rest of the egg mixture into the chocolate. Pour into prepared ramekins. Bake for 20 minutes. Cool completely, then refrigerate for at least 1 hour before adding ice cream.

Place ¼ cup of ice cream inside each ramekin, smoothing out top. Cover with plastic wrap and freeze.

(continued on next page)

FOR THE COCONUT ICE CREAM

2½ cups heavy cream

½ cup water

8 large egg yolks

3 tablespoons SomerSweet

2 tablespoons coconut extract

FOR THE CRUST

2 (4.9-ounce) SomerSweet Dark Chocolate Baking Bars (60 squares), chopped

3 ounces unsweetened baking chocolate, chopped

12 tablespoons (1½ sticks) unsalted butter

5 large eggs at room temperature

1 tablespoon SomerSweet

FOR THE MERINGUE

4 egg whites

2 teaspoons SomerSweet

½ teaspoon vanilla extract

SUGAR SUBSTITUTIONS
ice cream: ¾ cup sugar
crust: ¼ cup sugar
        10 ounces dark chocolate
meringue: 1 cup sugar

Preheat oven to 400°. Beat the egg whites in a mixer until soft peaks form. Add the SomerSweet and vanilla and beat until stiff peaks form. Dollop on top of the frozen ice cream. Place in the hot oven for 5 minutes, or until the meringue is golden brown. Cool for 5 minutes. Serve within 5 minutes.

SOMERSIZE COFFEE ICE CREAM

ALMOST LEVEL ONE   Makes 1 quart

3 cups heavy cream
5 large egg yolks, lightly
    beaten
3 tablespoons instant
    decaf coffee granules
3 tablespoons plus 2
    teaspoons SomerSweet
1 teaspoon vanilla extract
1 cup half-and-half

SUGAR SUBSTITUTIONS
1 cup sugar

This rich, wonderful ice cream is used in my Mocha Ice Cream Roll (page 57); of course, it's also fabulous all on its own.

Heat 2 cups of the cream (reserving 1 cup) in a small saucepan over low until small bubbles appear around outer edge. (If you use an instant-read thermometer, the temperature of the cream should read about 120°.) Remove from heat.

Place the yolks into the top of a double boiler over gently simmering water. Pour half of the hot cream over the egg yolks, stirring constantly. Cook until the mixture thickens slightly, about 4 minutes, or until a thermometer inserted into the mixture reads 160°. Add decaf coffee granules, SomerSweet, and vanilla. Whisk until the coffee has dissolved. Stir in the remaining 1 cup cream and the half-and-half. Refrigerate for 30 minutes. Freeze in an ice cream maker according to manufacturer's directions.

FRENCH VANILLA ICE CREAM

PRO/FATS—LEVEL ONE   Makes 1¹/₂ pints

Vanilla is a taste from my childhood. There were only three flavors then, and vanilla was my favorite. For the best French vanilla ice cream, use a real vanilla bean. To scrape it, split the vanilla bean lengthwise with the tip of a small, sharp knife. Scrape out the little black seeds with the knife and drip them right into the cream. Throw the pods in, too. Of course, you can also use my packaged Somersize Vanilla Bean Ice Cream Mix instead of this recipe; then all of the scraping is done for you.

2¹/₂ cups heavy cream
¹/₂ cup water
8 large egg yolks
2 whole vanilla beans, scraped, or 1 tablespoon vanilla extract
2 tablespoons SomerSweet

SUGAR SUBSTITUTIONS
³/₄ cup sugar

Pour the cream and water into a saucepan. Heat until hot, but not boiling. Remove from heat.

Place the egg yolks into a bowl. Whisk for 2 to 3 minutes, or until egg yolks are pale yellow. Pour the cream mixture over yolks, stirring constantly. Return to low heat, stirring constantly, until mixture thickens and coats the back of a spoon. Do not let mixture boil. Add scraped vanilla seeds and pods (or vanilla extract) and SomerSweet and stir. Cover surface of custard with plastic wrap. Cool to room temperature. Chill the custard for at least 2 hours or overnight. Remove the vanilla bean pods. Pour the mixture into an ice cream maker and freeze according to manufacturer's directions.

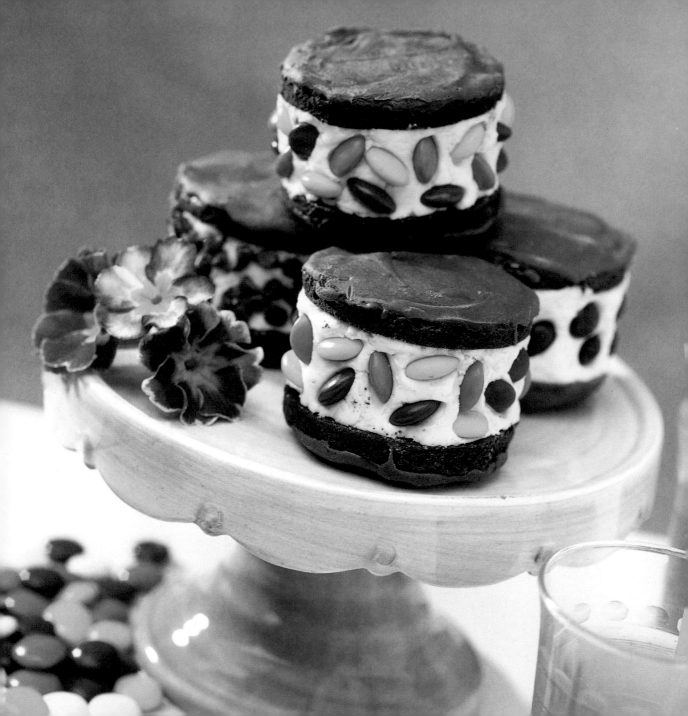

ICE CREAM SANDWICHES

ALMOST LEVEL ONE   **Makes 4 servings**

My grandchildren love these Ice Cream Sandwiches and so do I. Make them a special treat by adding my SomerSweet Zannies, Chocolate Chips, or Chocolate Covered Espresso Beans. No refined sugars—can you believe it?

Preheat oven to 350°. Butter a 9 × 13-inch cake pan. Dust with 1 tablespoon of the cocoa powder to prevent cake from sticking to pan. Set aside.

Melt the butter in a small, heavy saucepan over low heat. Add one of the chopped chocolate bars (reserving the other) and stir continuously until chocolate has melted and mixture is smooth. Remove from heat and set aside.

Place the eggs into a large bowl. Beat with an electric mixer until frothy, about 1 minute. Add the remaining cocoa powder, the SomerSweet, and vanilla and beat for another minute. Mixture will be thick. Slowly pour in melted chocolate while continuing to beat at low speed. Increase speed to medium and keep beating until mixture is smooth, about 30 seconds. Spread mixture evenly in prepared pan. Bake for 13 minutes. Allow to cool before cutting into 2½-inch circles with a round cookie cutter (or an empty SomerSweet can).

Melt the remaining chopped chocolate bar in a microwave or double boiler, stirring until chocolate is melted and smooth. Dip the outside of each cookie into melted chocolate. Allow excess to drip off. Place on a baking sheet lined with waxed paper. Freeze until chocolate has set.

TO ASSEMBLE SANDWICHES

Line a metal or plastic ⅓-cup round measuring cup with plastic wrap. Pack the measuring cup with ice cream. Place one cookie on top of the ice cream. Invert the measuring cup and remove the plastic wrap. Place another cookie on top. Roll ice cream edge in SomerSweet Zannies, Chocolate Chips, or Espresso Beans. Repeat with remaining cookies and ice cream. Freeze until the ice cream has set, then wrap tightly in plastic wrap and aluminum foil (to prevent freezer burn) and freeze for at least 4 hours, or overnight.

½ cup unsweetened cocoa powder

6 tablespoons (¾ stick) butter

2 (4.9-ounce) SomerSweet Milk Chocolate Baking Bars (60 squares), chopped

3 large eggs

2 tablespoons SomerSweet

1 teaspoon vanilla extract

1⅓ cups French Vanilla Ice Cream (page 35)

SomerSweet Zannies; SomerSweet Chocolate Chips; or SomerSweet Chocolate Covered Espresso Beans, for garnish

SUGAR SUBSTITUTIONS
¼ cup sugar
10 ounces dark chocolate

37

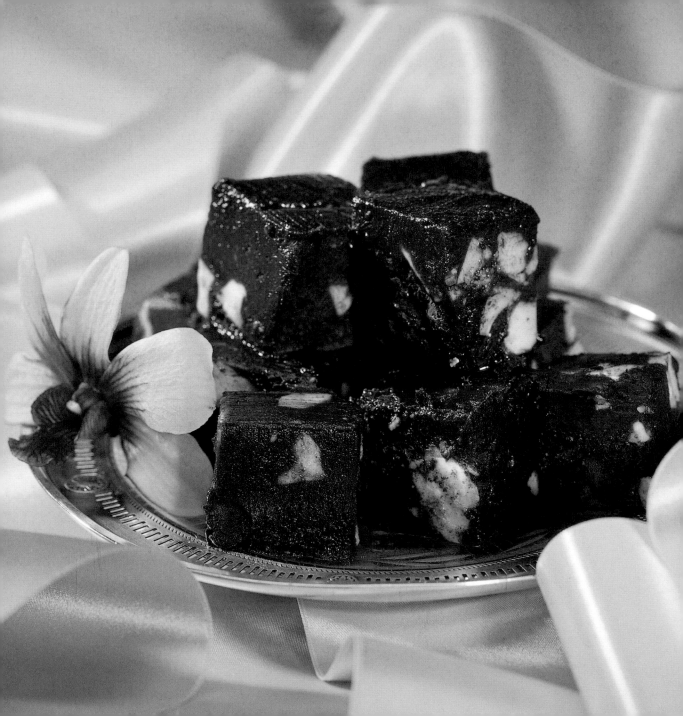

EASY WHITE CHOCOLATE CHUNK ICE BOX FUDGE

ALMOST LEVEL ONE   **Makes 30 pieces**

Gooey, yummy fudge has to be one of the ultimate sinful pleasures. This recipe is still the ultimate pleasure, but it's not sinful since it's made with SomerSweet.

Line a 9 × 5-inch loaf pan with a double layer of plastic wrap, allowing a few inches to overhang at each end. Set aside.

Heat the cream in a small saucepan over medium. When bubbles appear around edges, remove the pan from the heat. Add the milk chocolate and unsweetened chocolate to the cream. Stir until the chocolate has melted and the mixture is smooth.

Remove the lid and heat the caramel sauce for 20 seconds in the microwave. Pour into the chocolate mixture and stir well. Let cool to room temperature. (If it is too warm it will melt the white chocolate pieces.)

Stir the white chocolate pieces into the chocolate mixture. Pour into prepared pan. Chill overnight or until firm. Using overhanging plastic as handles, lift the fudge out of the pan. Peel off the plastic wrap. Let the fudge sit for 10 minutes to soften slightly before cutting into 1-inch pieces. Store refrigerated in an airtight container or wrap well and freeze for up to 3 months.

1 cup heavy cream

2 (4.9-ounce) SomerSweet Milk or Dark Chocolate Baking Bars (60 squares), chopped

4 ounces unsweetened baking chocolate, chopped

1 (7.4-ounce) jar Somersize Caramel Sauce

2.5 ounces, or $1/2$ SomerSweet White Chocolate Baking Bar (15 squares), cut into $1/4$-inch pieces and chilled

SUGAR SUBSTITUTIONS
10 ounces dark chocolate

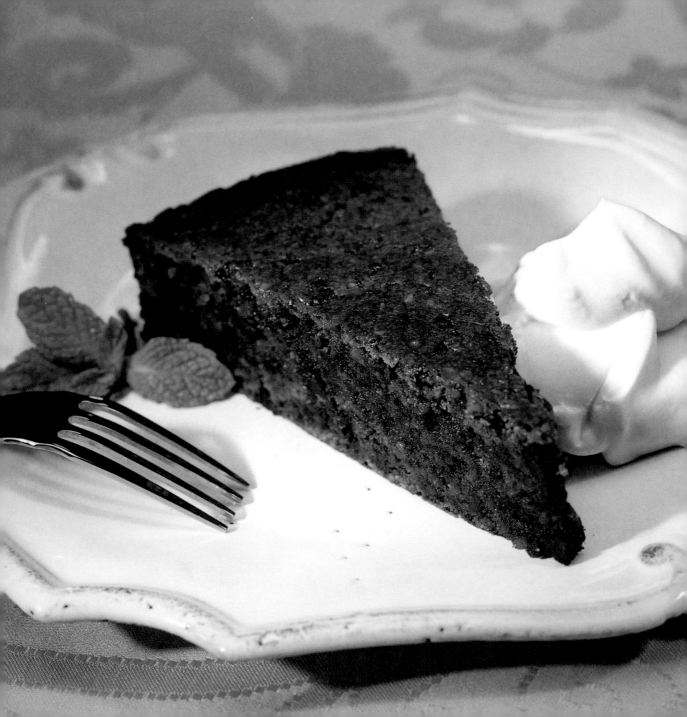

CHOCOLATE ALMOND TORTE

LEVEL TWO   **Makes 12 servings**

This tasty recipe first appeared in *Get Skinny on Fabulous Food.* Now it's even better (and easier) using SomerSweet Baking Bars. The almonds create a slight imbalance because of the small addition of carbohydrates in nuts. It's a perfect Level Two dessert.

Preheat oven to 400°. Butter an 8-inch springform pan. Line bottom with waxed or parchment paper. Butter top of waxed paper and set aside.

Coarsely grind the almonds with 1 tablespoon SomerSweet in a food processor. Add the chocolate and process until chocolate and almonds are finely ground. Set aside.

Cream the butter and remaining 2 tablespoons SomerSweet with an electric mixer until light and pale in color. Add the yolks one by one, beating between each addition. Add the chocolate mixture. Stir until combined. Set aside.

In a separate bowl beat the egg whites until they form soft peaks. Using a rubber spatula, gently fold a quarter of the egg whites into the chocolate mixture. Fold the chocolate mixture back into the remaining egg whites. Pour the batter into the prepared pan and bake for 45 minutes or until set.

Serve with Perfectly Whipped Cream or Crème Anglaise.

1¹/₂ cups (6 ounces) whole
    blanched almonds
3 tablespoons SomerSweet
2 (4.9-ounce) SomerSweet
    Dark Chocolate Baking Bars
    (60 squares), chopped
1 cup (2 sticks) unsalted
    butter at room temperature
6 large eggs, separated
Perfectly Whipped Cream
    (page 23) or Crème
    Anglaise (page 49)

SUGAR SUBSTITUTIONS
¹/₂ cup sugar
10 ounces dark chocolate

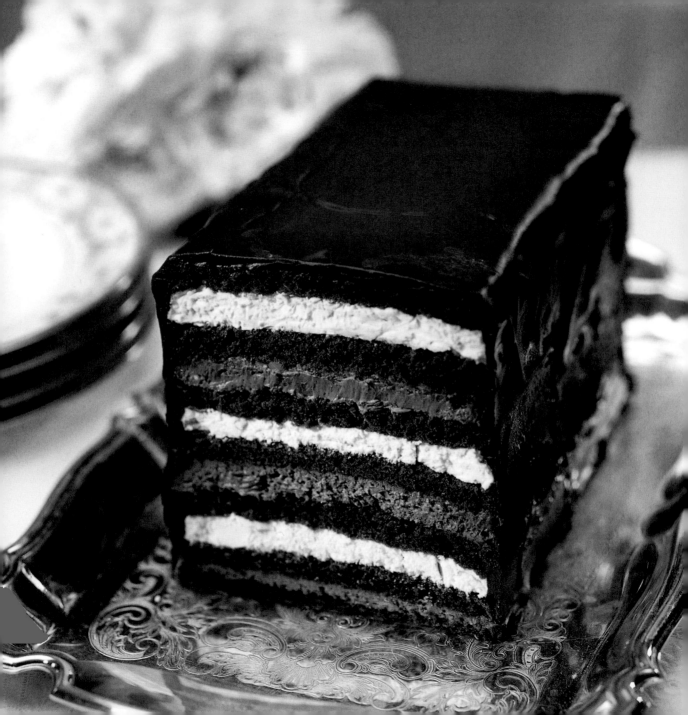

DOBOS TORTE

ALMOST LEVEL ONE   Makes 12 servings

Don't get overwhelmed by this one. It may seem daunting, but it's really quite easy. This spectacular torte is named for its creator, Austrian chef Josef Dobos. The traditional version has nine extra-thin layers of cake with buttercream in between. The time it takes is well worth it for a special occasion. It feeds a lot of people and the leftovers freeze beautifully. Simply bring back to room temperature before serving.

Beat the cream cheese with an electric mixer until light and fluffy, about 5 minutes. Add 1½ cups sour cream and the SomerSweet. Mix until smooth. Slowly add the heavy cream, beating constantly. Divide the mixture between two bowls. Fold half of the grated white chocolate into one bowl. Set aside.

Melt half of the dark chocolate in a microwave, stirring every 30 seconds, until chocolate is melted and smooth. Carefully fold the melted chocolate into the other bowl of cream cheese mixture. Cover and chill both bowls for at least 1 hour.

TO ASSEMBLE CAKE

Cut each cake into four equal pieces, measuring about 9 × 3 inches, so that you have eight cake layers total. Place a layer of cake on a cooling rack set on top of a baking sheet. Spread a third of the dark filling on top of the cake. Place another cake layer on top. Spread a third of the white filling on top. Put another cake layer on top of the white filling. Keep repeating layers until you have used all the filling and cake layers. It's okay if you have one cake layer left—eat it as a snack. Smooth the sides with a spatula. Refrigerate for 1 hour.

Meanwhile, make the ganache. Melt the rest of the white chocolate and dark chocolate, the unsweetened chocolate, and butter in the top of a double boiler over gently simmering water. Stir until the chocolate has melted and the mixture is smooth. Stir in the remaining 1 tablespoon sour cream. Cover until ready to use.

(continued on next page)

2 (8-ounce) packages cream cheese at room temperature
1½ cups plus 1 tablespoon sour cream
¼ cup SomerSweet
½ cup heavy cream
1 (4.9-ounce) SomerSweet White Chocolate Baking Bar (30 squares), grated
1 (4.9-ounce) SomerSweet Dark Chocolate Baking Bar (30 squares), chopped
1 recipe Chocolate Cake for Dobos Torte (page 44)
1 ounce unsweetened baking chocolate, chopped
½ cup (1 stick) unsalted butter

SUGAR SUBSTITUTIONS
¾ cup sugar
5 ounces white chocolate
5 ounces dark chocolate

When the cake has chilled for an hour, pour ¼ cup ganache into a small bowl. (If ganache has hardened, simply reheat and stir for a few moments.) Using a pastry brush, brush the cake all over with a thin layer of ganache. (This will help make the final coating smooth.) Refrigerate for 30 minutes. Pour the remaining ganache over the entire cake, letting it drip down and coat the sides. Use a pastry brush to spread ganache over any missed areas. Refrigerate the cake until the ganache has set, at least 30 minutes. Carefully transfer from the rack to a serving platter and cut into ¾-inch slices.

CHOCOLATE CAKE FOR DOBOS TORTE

ALMOST LEVEL ONE   **Makes 2 layers**

This delicious cake has no flour at all! It's a great base for many Almost Level One desserts.

1 cup plus 1 tablespoon unsweetened cocoa powder

12 tablespoons (1½ sticks) unsalted butter

2 (4.9-ounce) SomerSweet Dark Chocolate Baking Bars (60 squares), chopped

6 large eggs

¼ cup SomerSweet

2 teaspoons vanilla extract

SUGAR SUBSTITUTIONS
¾ cup sugar
10 ounces dark chocolate

Preheat oven to 350°. Butter two 9 × 13-inch baking or cake pans. Dust with 1 tablespoon cocoa powder to prevent cake from sticking to pan. Set aside.

Melt the butter in a small, heavy saucepan over low heat. Add the chocolate and stir continuously until chocolate has melted and mixture is smooth. Remove from heat and set aside.

In the bowl of an electric mixer, beat the eggs until frothy, about 1 minute. Add the remaining 1 cup cocoa powder, the SomerSweet, and vanilla and beat for another minute. Mixture will be thick. Slowly add the melted chocolate mixture while continuing to beat at low speed. Increase the speed to medium and continue beating until the mixture is smooth, about 30 seconds. Spread the batter evenly into the prepared pans. Bake for 15 minutes. Allow to cool before removing carefully from baking pans.

CHOCOLATE TRUFFLE FROSTING

ALMOST LEVEL ONE Makes 2 cups

This is simply the richest chocolate frosting ever. It's perfect for filling and frosting your fantastic cake.

Bring the coffee granules and cream to a boil in a medium saucepan. Simmer gently for 2 minutes. Remove from the heat and set aside.

Place both chocolates and the SomerSweet into a food processor. Pulse until the chocolate is finely ground. With the machine running, pour the hot cream mixture into the ground chocolate. Add the vanilla and eggs, and blend until smooth. Pour the mixture into a double boiler and set over gently simmering water. Cook for 2 to 3 minutes, stirring constantly, until the frosting is very warm to the touch. Let frosting cool in the refrigerator, stirring occasionally, until it becomes stiff enough to spread, about 30 minutes. (If frosting chills too long it will become very stiff. Simply let it sit at room temperature until the proper consistency is reached.)

$1/4$ cup decaf coffee granules

2 cups heavy cream

4 (4.9-ounce) SomerSweet Milk Chocolate Baking Bars (120 squares), chopped

4 ounces unsweetened baking chocolate, chopped

$1/4$ cup SomerSweet

1 tablespoon vanilla extract

4 large eggs at room temperature

SUGAR SUBSTITUTIONS
$1/2$ cup sugar
20 ounces dark chocolate

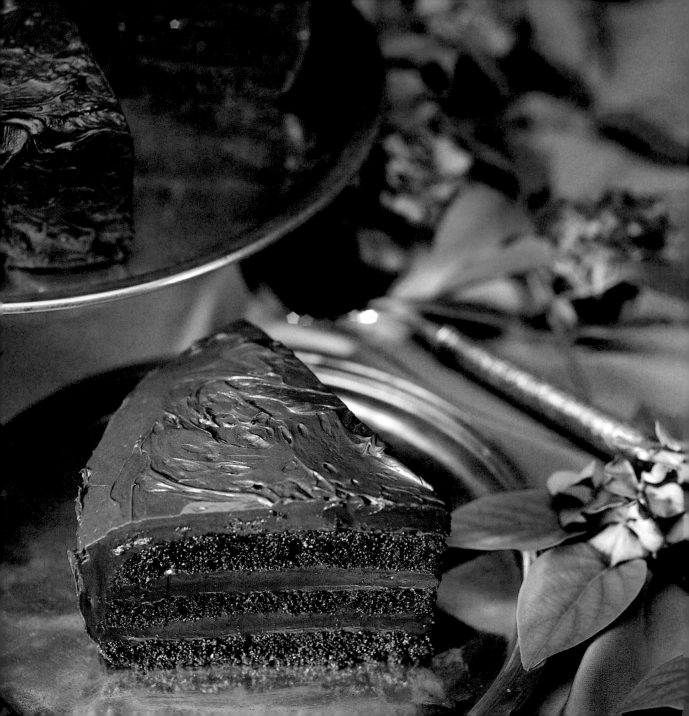

CHOCOLATE BLACKOUT CAKE

LEVEL TWO   Makes 12 servings

What chocolate book would be complete without a fabulous chocolate cake? This dense, rich cake makes the best birthday cake ever! This is a Level Two cake because of the addition of whole wheat flour. Get the candles and make a wish! The white whole wheat flour makes a lighter cake, which I prefer.

Preheat oven to 350°. Butter the bottom and sides of a 9-inch springform pan. Cut a 9-inch circle of waxed or parchment paper and place into the bottom of the pan. Butter top of waxed paper and set aside.

Melt the chocolates and butter together in a double boiler over gently simmering water. Stir until chocolate is melted and smooth. Remove from the heat and allow mixture to cool slightly. Sift together the flour and baking soda and set aside.

Meanwhile, separate the eggs and beat the whites until soft peaks form. Add the SomerSweet and beat for another minute. Set aside. In another bowl, beat the yolks until foamy, about 5 minutes. Carefully fold a third of the flour mixture into the yolks. Carefully fold a third of the chocolate mixture into the yolks. Repeat until all the flour and chocolate are incorporated. Fold the yolk mixture into the egg whites. Pour into the prepared pan.

Bake for 35 to 40 minutes or until cake is set in the center. Allow to sit at room temperature for 20 minutes before refrigerating. Chill completely before slicing into three layers. Frost the two inside layers thickly with half of the Chocolate Truffle Frosting. Assemble the layers and spread the remaining frosting on the top and sides of the cake.

14.4 ounces, or 4$\frac{1}{2}$ SomerSweet Dark Chocolate Baking Bars (135 squares), chopped

6 ounces unsweetened baking chocolate, chopped

1$\frac{1}{2}$ cups (3 sticks) plus 3 tablespoons unsalted butter

1$\frac{1}{2}$ cups 100% white whole wheat flour (or whole wheat pastry flour)

$\frac{3}{4}$ teaspoon baking soda

12 large eggs at room temperature

3 tablespoons SomerSweet

1 recipe Chocolate Truffle Frosting (page 45)

SUGAR SUBSTITUTIONS
1 cup sugar
1$\frac{1}{2}$ pounds dark chocolate

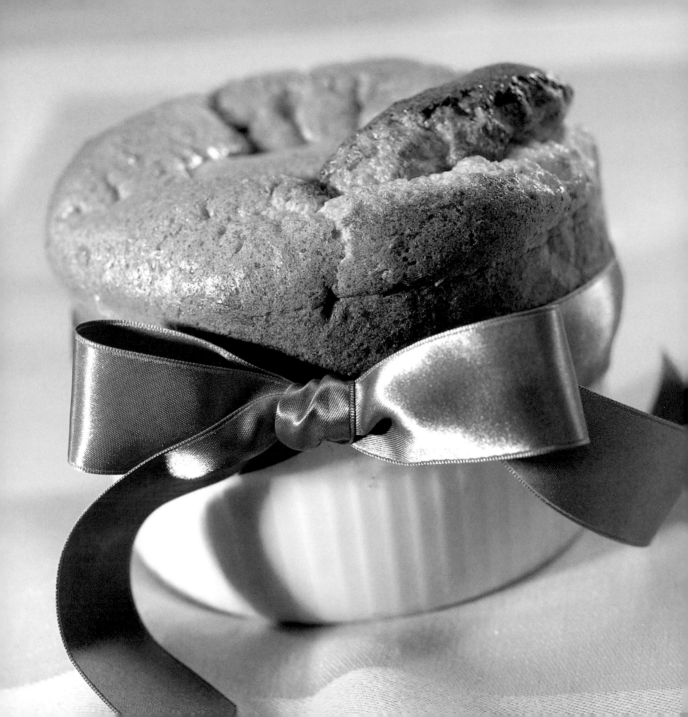

WHITE CHOCOLATE SOUFFLÉ

ALMOST LEVEL ONE   **Makes 4 servings**

This is yummy! Don't be afraid of soufflés—this one is foolproof! It's as light and fluffy as a cloud. With one bite you'll think you've died and gone to heaven! As a variation, serve it with my Somersize Caramel or Triple Hot Fudge Sauce or Raspberry Jam.

Preheat oven to 350°. Butter a 1-quart soufflé dish and set aside.

Bring the cream to a boil in a medium saucepan. Remove immediately from heat. Add the chopped chocolate and SomerSweet to the hot cream and stir until the chocolate is melted and smooth. Set aside.

Beat the egg yolks in an electric mixer until thick and pale in color, about 5 minutes. Add the vanilla. Slowly add the cream mixture, stirring constantly. Set aside.

Beat the egg whites with an electric mixer until they form stiff peaks. Fold the egg whites into the yolk mixture. Pour into the prepared soufflé dish. Bake in the center of the oven for 30 minutes, or until the top is golden brown. While still hot, make a hole in the center and pour in Crème Anglaise.

1¾ cups heavy cream
6.14 ounces, or 1½
    SomerSweet White
    Chocolate Baking Bars
    (45 squares), chopped
4 teaspoons SomerSweet
3 large eggs, separated
1 teaspoon vanilla extract
1 recipe Crème Anglaise
    (see below)

SUGAR SUBSTITUTIONS
½ cup sugar
10 ounces white chocolate

CRÈME ANGLAISE
PRO/FATS—LEVEL ONE   **Makes 2¼ cups**

Crème Anglaise is a thin, rich custard sauce that is divine on nearly any dessert.

Whisk the egg yolks and vanilla in a bowl and set aside. Heat the cream over medium until hot, but not boiling. Remove the cream from the heat and add the SomerSweet. Pour cream over the egg yolks, whisking constantly. Return to the saucepan and heat on low, whisking constantly until mixture thickens and coats the back of a spoon. Serve warm or cover and refrigerate until ready to use.

6 large egg yolks
1¾ teaspoons vanilla extract
2 cups heavy cream
2¼ teaspoons SomerSweet

SUGAR SUBSTITUTIONS
3 tablespoons sugar

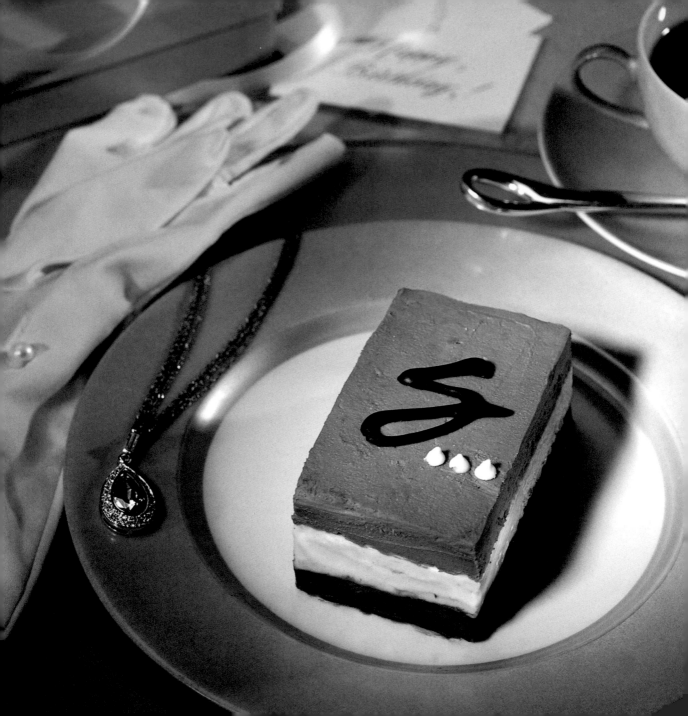

TRIPLE CHOCOLATE TERRINE

ALMOST LEVEL ONE   **Makes 12 servings**

Hmm . . . white chocolate, milk chocolate, dark chocolate—so hard to decide! Now you don't have to with this fabulous Triple Chocolate Terrine. Feel free to decorate with your own chocolate initial or design. This decadent dessert makes enough for a party and, if wrapped and refrigerated, will keep for up to five days.

Line a 9 × 5-inch loaf pan with plastic wrap, allowing plastic wrap to over-hang sides of pan by at least 3 inches. Set aside.

Beat the cream cheese and SomerSweet together until smooth. Add vanilla and stir well.

In a separate bowl, beat the cream with an electric mixer until stiff. Care-fully fold the cream cheese mixture into the whipped cream. Set aside.

Place each type of chocolate into a separate microwave-safe bowl. Micro-wave each in 30-second intervals, stirring in between, until all the chocolate is melted and smooth. Carefully fold a third of the cream mixture into each of the three bowls of melted chocolate. Spread the dark chocolate mixture into the bottom of the prepared loaf pan. Tap pan on counter to even out the layer. Spread the white chocolate mixture evenly over the dark chocolate layer. Spoon the milk chocolate layer on top of the white chocolate layer. Cover with plastic wrap and refrigerate overnight. To serve, remove the outer plastic wrap, then invert loaf pan onto a serving plate. Remove the remaining plastic wrap. Cut into ¾-inch slices.

To make decorations, pipe melted chocolate onto waxed paper in desired design. Freeze for about a minute. Carefully remove from waxed paper and transfer to terrine.

---

2 (8-ounce) packages cream cheese at room temperature
1 tablespoon SomerSweet
2 teaspoons vanilla extract
1¼ cups whipping cream
1 (4.9-ounce) SomerSweet Dark Chocolate Baking Bar (30 squares), chopped
1 (4.9-ounce) SomerSweet Milk Chocolate Baking Bar (30 squares), chopped
1 (4.9-ounce) SomerSweet White Chocolate Baking Bar (30 squares), chopped

SUGAR SUBSTITUTIONS
¼ cup sugar
5 ounces dark chocolate
5 ounces milk chocolate
5 ounces white chocolate

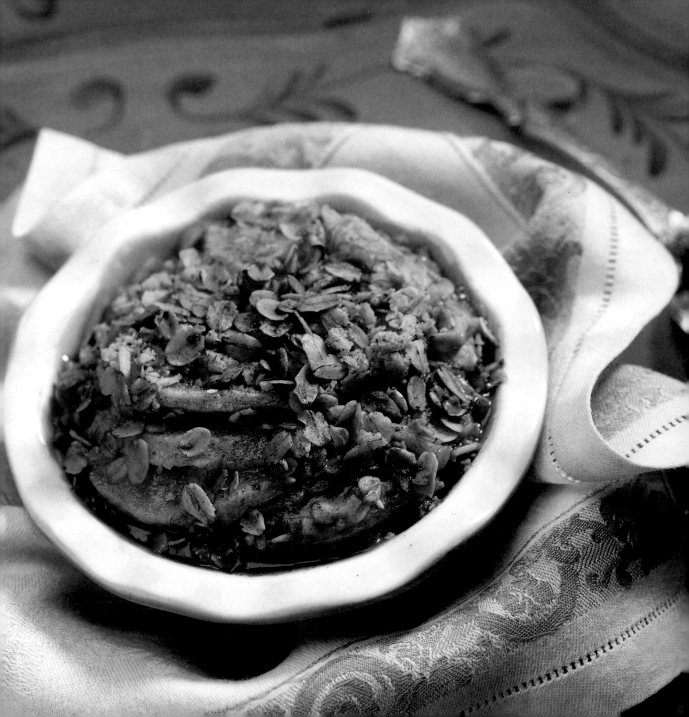

PEAR COBBLER WITH CHOCOLATE CRUMBLE TOPPING

LEVEL TWO   **Makes 6 servings**

A ripe pear, rolled oats, butter, cinnamon, and a sprinkle of chocolate—this must be heaven! Do I have to say it? Serve this with my warm Somersize Pear Cinnamon Caramel Sauce (available at SuzanneSomers.com).

TO MAKE FILLING

Preheat oven to 375°. Butter a 13×9-inch baking dish and set aside. Combine the pear slices, lemon juice, and almond extract in a large bowl. Add the SomerSweet and flour and toss to combine. Pour the filling into the prepared baking dish. Set aside.

TO MAKE CRUMBLE TOPPING

Mix the flour, oats, SomerSweet, and cinnamon in a medium bowl. Add the butter and rub in with your fingers until moist clumps form. Mix in the chopped chocolate. Set aside.

Sprinkle the topping over the pear mixture. Bake until the topping is golden brown, 25 to 30 minutes. Cool at least 20 minutes before serving. Serve warm or at room temperature.

FOR THE FILLING

3 pounds ripe pears, peeled, cored, and cut into 1/4-inch-thick slices, or 2 pounds frozen sliced pears, thawed and drained

1 tablespoon lemon juice

1 1/2 teaspoons almond extract

2 tablespoons SomerSweet

1 1/2 tablespoons 100% white whole wheat flour (or whole wheat pastry flour)

FOR THE TOPPING

1/2 cup 100% white whole wheat flour

2/3 cup old-fashioned rolled oats

2 tablespoons SomerSweet

1 teaspoon cinnamon

4 tablespoons (1/2 stick) unsalted butter, cut into 1/4-inch pieces

1 (4.9-ounce) SomerSweet Milk Chocolate Baking Bar (30 squares), chopped into 1/4-inch pieces

SUGAR SUBSTITUTIONS
filling: 1/2 cup sugar
topping: 1/4 cup sugar
5 ounces dark chocolate

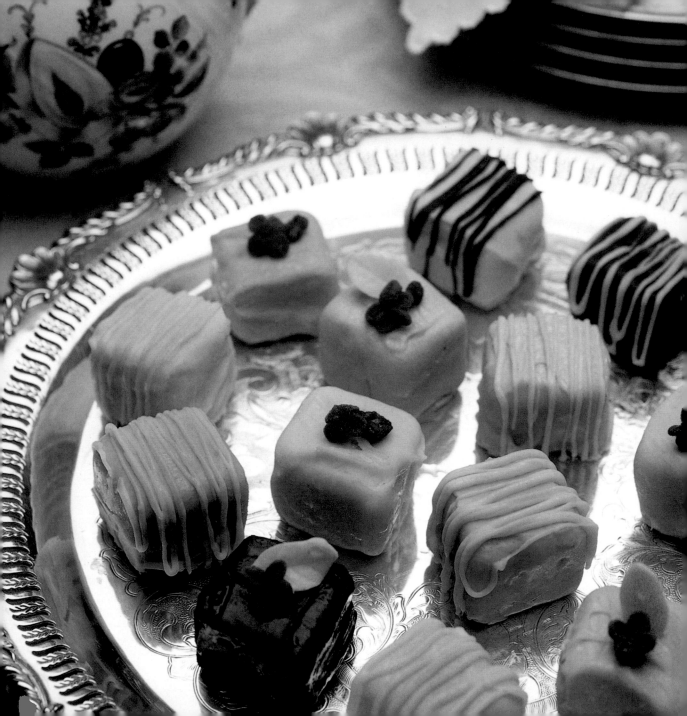

CHOCOLATE CHEESECAKE PETIT FOURS

ALMOST LEVEL ONE   **Makes 40 petit fours**

Here is my version of fancy petit fours as you'd find them in expensive bakeries. These cream-cheesy treats are bite size and perfect for dessert. Keep them in the freezer for whenever you want a sweet treat. I make them in a variety of dark, milk, and white chocolate. Add a few drops of food coloring to the white chocolate to create a palette to match your table. The ones I made are decorated with candied violets and lilacs.

Preheat oven to 350°. Line the bottom of a 9-inch springform pan (2½ inches deep) or cake pan with waxed paper. Grease the bottom and sides with butter. Wrap the outside with a double layer of foil to prevent seepage. Set aside.

In a large bowl, beat the cream cheese with an electric mixer until fluffy. Add the SomerSweet and beat for another minute. Add the eggs one at a time, beating well to combine after each addition. Add the vanilla and beat until smooth. Pour the batter into the prepared pan. Set the pan inside a large roasting pan or baking dish. Place into the oven and pour very hot water into the roasting pan to reach halfway up the sides of the springform pan. Bake for 1 hour. Turn off the heat without opening the door and allow the cake to cool in the oven for 1 hour more. Remove the cake from the oven and place onto a cooling rack for another hour. Cover with plastic wrap and refrigerate overnight.

Unmold the cheesecake onto a work surface. Carefully peel away the waxed paper. Cut the cheesecake into forty 1-inch squares using a knife warmed under hot running water. Set aside.

Melt the chocolate bars and butter in a double boiler or microwave. Stir until the mixture is smooth. Drop each cheesecake square into the melted chocolate. Using a fork, lift the squares out of the chocolate, allowing excess chocolate to drip off. Place on a cookie sheet lined with waxed or parchment paper. Store refrigerated in an airtight container for at least 2 hours or until the chocolate has hardened. These will keep for up to a week and can be frozen for up to 6 months.

3 (8-ounce) packages cream cheese at room temperature
2 tablespoons SomerSweet
3 large eggs at room temperature
1 teaspoon vanilla extract
2 (4.9-ounce) SomerSweet White, Milk, or Dark Chocolate Baking Bars (60 squares)
3 tablespoons unsalted butter

SUGAR SUBSTITUTIONS
½ cup sugar
10 ounces dark chocolate

FOR A PRESENTATION VARIATION
Decorate by melting a little of my SomerSweet White Chocolate Baking Bar and dipping a fork into it, allowing the chocolate to drizzle off onto the tops of the petit fours. You can also melt my white chocolate baking bar and add food coloring for pastel petit fours. Decorate with my SomerSweet Rose Petals (page 69), Chocolate Leaves (page 85), or Lemon and Orange Slices (page 69).

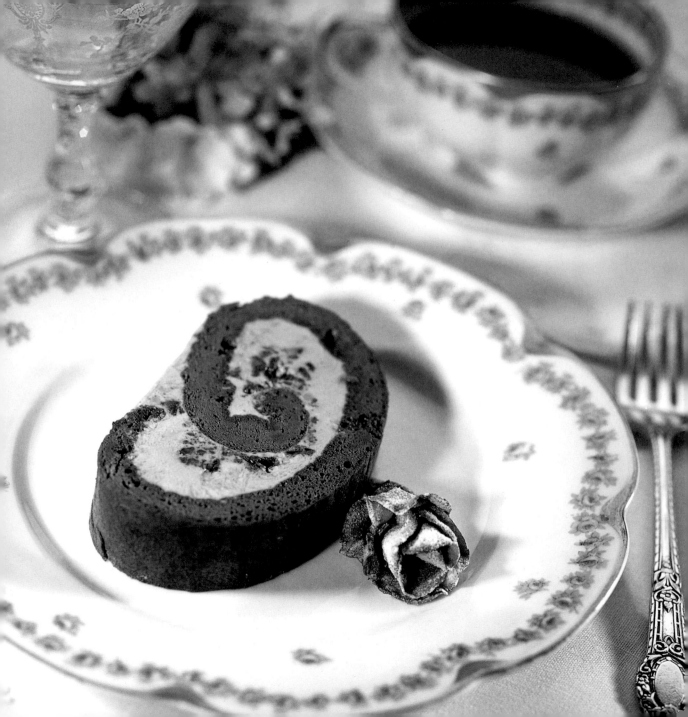

MOCHA ICE CREAM ROLL

ALMOST LEVEL ONE   Makes 8–10 servings

You can make this recipe even easier by whipping up the ice cream with my Somersize Coffee Ice Cream Mix. One slice of this roll makes an elegant dessert fit for company. Directions for SomerSweet Rose Petals are on page 69.

Preheat oven to 300°. Line a nonstick 9×13-inch jellyroll or cake pan with waxed or parchment paper. Butter the waxed paper and set aside.

With an electric mixer, beat together the egg yolks, mayonnaise, cream, cocoa powder, vanilla, salt, and SomerSweet until smooth. Set aside.

In another bowl, beat the egg whites until very stiff. Fold the yolk mixture into the egg whites. Spread in the jellyroll pan and bake for 30 to 35 minutes or until set. Let cool a few minutes before handling. Using a spatula, loosen the edges of the cake. Invert the cake onto a clean work surface. While cake is still warm, lay a piece of plastic wrap over its surface. Place a clean kitchen towel on top of the plastic wrap. Roll cake up like a jellyroll. Set aside and allow cake to cool completely before assembling.

To assemble, unroll the cooled cake. Spread the surface evenly with softened ice cream. Sprinkle the ice cream with the chopped chocolate. Carefully push the chocolate pieces into the ice cream, then reroll the cake. It's okay if cake cracks somewhat. Place cake, seam side down, on a clean baking pan. Freeze for 2 hours. Wrap in plastic wrap, then in aluminum foil, and freeze overnight. To serve, cut into 1-inch slices. Can be frozen for up to 6 months.

4 large egg yolks

¼ cup mayonnaise

2 tablespoons heavy cream

¼ cup unsweetened cocoa powder

1 teaspoon vanilla extract

Pinch salt

1 tablespoon SomerSweet

6 large egg whites at room temperature

2 cups Somersize Coffee Ice Cream (page 34), softened

2.5 ounces or ½ SomerSweet Dark or Milk Chocolate Baking Bar (15 squares), chopped into ¼-inch pieces

SUGAR SUBSTITUTIONS
3 tablespoons sugar
3 ounces dark chocolate

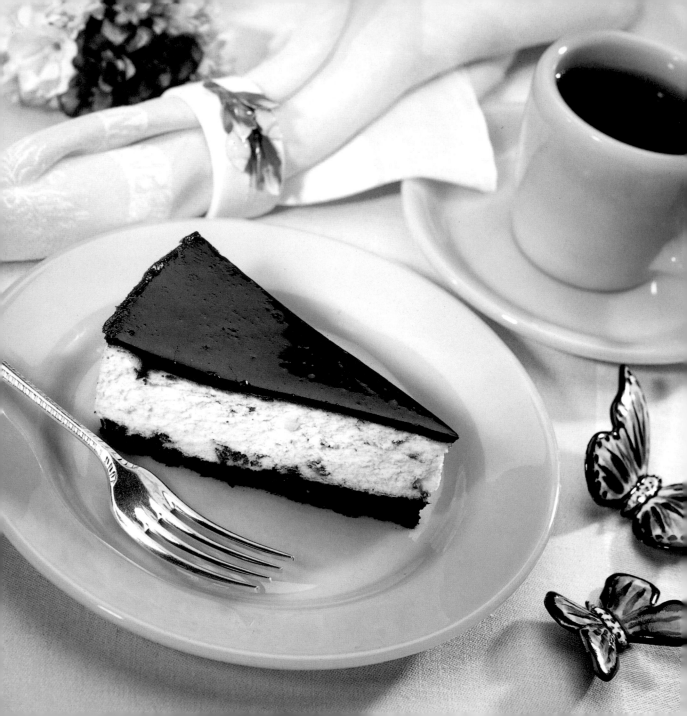

PEPPERMINT CHEESECAKE WITH CHOCOLATE CRUST

ALMOST LEVEL ONE   **Makes 12 servings**

This great cheesecake has an unexpected twist of mint. To make the topping super easy, pop open a jar of Somersize Chocolate Mint Hot Fudge Sauce.

TO MAKE CRUST

Preheat oven to 275°. Butter a 9-inch springform pan. Set aside.

Place the cocoa powder, baking soda, SomerSweet, and butter into a food processor. Pulse until mixture resembles cornmeal. Add the egg and vanilla and pulse until mixture forms pea-size pieces. Pour into prepared pan. Press into bottom of pan and set aside.

TO MAKE CHEESECAKE

In a large mixing bowl, beat the cream cheese and SomerSweet until light and fluffy. Add the eggs one at a time, beating well after each addition. Add the cream and peppermint extract. Mix until smooth. Pour filling into prepared pan and place in a roasting pan or baking dish. Place the roasting pan into the oven and pour very hot water into the roasting pan to reach halfway up the sides of the springform pan. Bake for 1 hour. Without opening the oven door, turn off the heat and leave cheesecake in the oven for an additional hour.

TO MAKE TOPPING

Meanwhile, make the chocolate topping by heating the cream in a small, heavy saucepan. When small bubbles appear around the edges, remove from the heat and stir in the chocolate. Continue stirring until the chocolate is melted and smooth. Pour over the cooled cheesecake. Refrigerate overnight. Run a warm knife around the edges of the cheesecake before releasing the spring. Transfer the cheesecake to a serving dish.

FOR THE CRUST

1 1/2 cups unsweetened cocoa powder
1/2 teaspoon baking soda
2 tablespoons plus 1 teaspoon SomerSweet
1/2 cup (1 stick) butter, chilled and cut into 1/2-inch pieces
1 large egg
1 teaspoon vanilla extract

FOR THE CHEESECAKE

3 (8-ounce) packages cream cheese at room temperature
2 tablespoons plus 1 teaspoon SomerSweet
4 large eggs
1 cup heavy cream
2 1/2 teaspoons pure peppermint extract

FOR THE TOPPING

1/2 cup heavy cream
1 (4.9-ounce) SomerSweet Dark or Milk Chocolate Baking Bar (30 squares), chopped

SUGAR SUBSTITUTIONS
crust: 1/4 cup sugar
cheesecake: 3/4 cup sugar
topping: 5 ounces dark chocolate

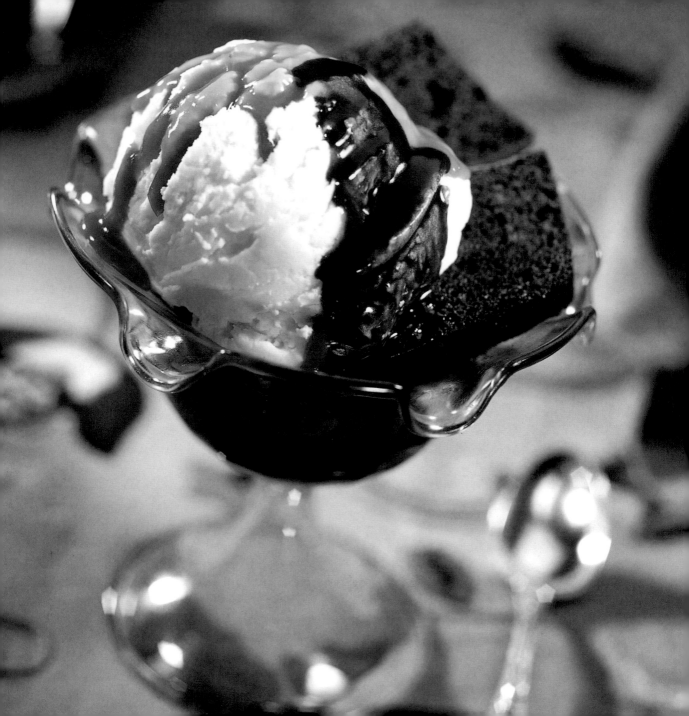

CARAMEL CHOCOLATE BROWNIE SUNDAES

LEVEL TWO   **Makes 4 servings**

Brownies, ice cream, caramel sauce, hot fudge, and whipped cream. Life is grand . . . so is dessert! Any one of these items would be considered Almost Level One. If you put them all together it probably topples into Level Two.

TO MAKE BROWNIES

Preheat oven to 400°. Line an 8-inch square baking pan with foil. Allow foil to overhang by a few inches. Butter foil and set pan aside.

Melt the chocolates and butter together in a double boiler over gently simmering water. Stir until chocolate is smooth. Remove from the heat and allow mixture to cool slightly.

Meanwhile, beat the eggs until pale and tripled in volume, 8 to 10 minutes (very important). Add the SomerSweet and beat for another minute. Mix one third of the egg mixture into the chocolate mixture. Carefully fold the rest of the egg mixture into the chocolate mixture. Pour into the prepared pan. Pour ½ cup caramel or fudge sauce on top of brownie batter and swirl in with a butter knife.

Bake for 30 minutes. Batter will not appear to be completely set. Cool for 15 minutes before lifting brownies out of pan by the foil handles. Carefully peel away foil. Cut brownies into 2½- to 3-inch squares (this will give you 9 brownies, so you will have 5 left over for snacking).

TO ASSEMBLE SUNDAES

Place one brownie in each of four dessert bowls. Top with a ½-cup scoop of French Vanilla Ice Cream. Drizzle with warmed caramel and fudge sauces.

FOR THE BROWNIES

2 (4.9-ounce) SomerSweet Dark Chocolate Baking Bars (60 squares), chopped

3 ounces unsweetened baking chocolate, chopped

12 tablespoons (1½ sticks) unsalted butter

5 large eggs at room temperature

1 tablespoon SomerSweet

½ cup Somersize Caramel or Triple Fudge Sauce, warmed

FOR THE SUNDAES

2 cups French Vanilla Ice Cream (page 35)

1 (7-ounce) jar Somersize Caramel Sauce, warmed

1 (7-ounce) jar Somersize Triple Hot Fudge Sauce, warmed

SUGAR SUBSTITUTIONS
3 tablespoons sugar
10 ounces dark chocolate

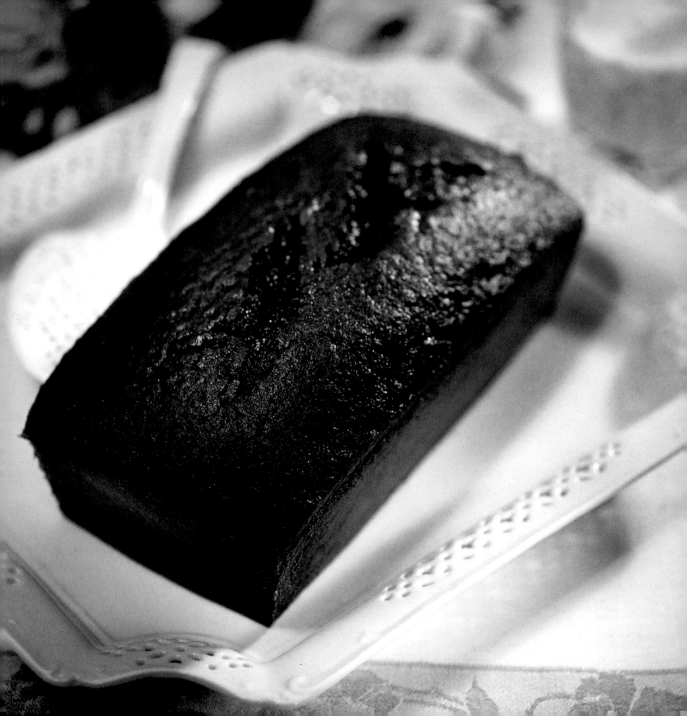

CHOCOLATE POUND CAKE

ALMOST LEVEL ONE   Makes 12 servings

I have always loved pound cake. Now that it's chocolate, there's even more reason to love it! Serve this with a drizzle of white chocolate glaze—just because you can! Powdered egg whites can be found at most natural food stores.

Preheat oven to 350°. Butter a 9 × 5-inch loaf pan. Set aside.

Melt half the chocolate and all the butter in a double boiler over gently simmering water. Stir until mixture is smooth. Pour into a medium bowl and stir in the eggs, vanilla, cream, and mayonnaise.

In a separate bowl, mix the cocoa powder, powdered egg whites, Somer-Sweet, and baking soda. Gradually stir the dry ingredients into the chocolate mixture.

Chop the remaining chocolate bar into ¼-inch pieces. Stir the chocolate pieces into the batter. Pour the batter into the prepared pan. Bake for 25 minutes. Allow the pound cake to cool completely. It is normal for pound cake to deflate somewhat during cooling. Keep cake refrigerated, then bring to room temperature before serving. Serve with a drizzle of White Chocolate Glaze.

WHITE CHOCOLATE GLAZE
ALMOST LEVEL ONE   Makes ⅓ cup

You can also use this glaze on my Chocolate Decadent Brownies (page 73) or drizzle it over the top of my Chocolate Blackout Cake (page 47).

Bring the cream to a simmer in a small, heavy saucepan. Remove from heat. Add the chocolate and vanilla and stir until chocolate has melted and glaze is smooth. Let cool for a few minutes before pouring.

---

1 (4.9-ounce) SomerSweet Dark or Milk Chocolate Baking Bar (30 squares)
½ cup (1 stick) unsalted butter, cut into ½-inch pieces
4 large eggs, lightly beaten
1 teaspoon vanilla extract
¼ cup heavy cream
1 cup mayonnaise
½ cup unsweetened cocoa powder
⅓ cup powdered egg whites
1 tablespoon plus 1 teaspoon SomerSweet
¼ teaspoon baking soda
1 recipe White Chocolate Glaze (see below)

SUGAR SUBSTITUTIONS
¾ cup sugar
5 ounces dark chocolate

3 tablespoons heavy cream
2.5 ounces or ½ SomerSweet White Chocolate Baking Bar (15 squares), chopped
½ teaspoon vanilla extract

SUGAR SUBSTITUTIONS
3 ounces white chocolate

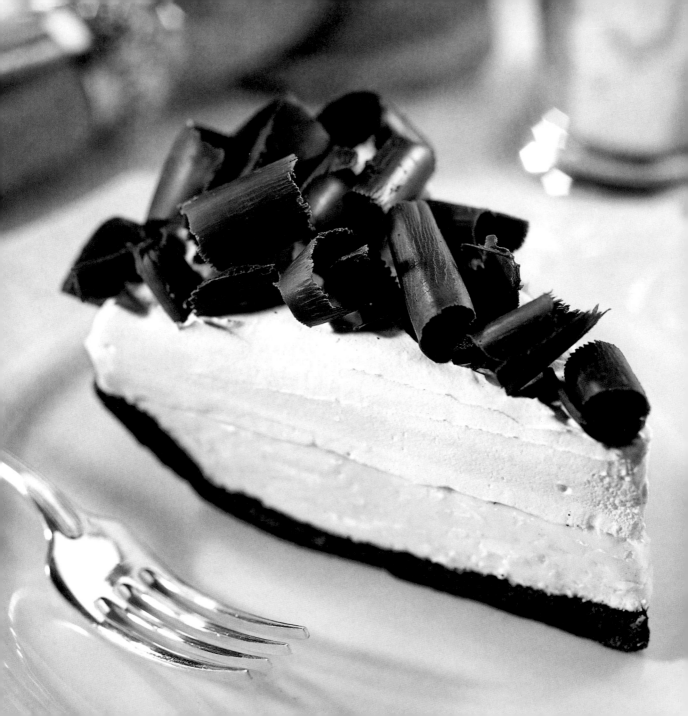

GRASSHOPPER PIE WITH CHOCOLATE CURLS

ALMOST LEVEL ONE   Makes 6–8 servings

This is for my son, Bruce, because as a boy, his favorite dessert was grasshopper pie. Now it is easier than ever by using a package of Somersize Mint Ice Cream for the filling. Plus, you can make the chocolate crust by combining a box of Somersize Flourless Chocolate Brownie mix with 1/2 stick cold butter. Pulse in a food processor until crumbly, then pour into a springform pan and bake at 350° for 10 minutes. Easy!

TO MAKE CRUST

Preheat oven to 275°. Butter a 9-inch glass pie plate and set aside.

Place the cocoa powder, baking soda, SomerSweet, and butter into a food processor. Pulse until the mixture resembles cornmeal. Add the egg and vanilla, and pulse until mixture forms pea-size pieces. Press into the bottom of the pie plate. Bake for 10 minutes. Allow to cool completely before filling.

TO MAKE ICE CREAM

Pour the cream and water into a heavy saucepan. Heat until hot, but not boiling. Remove from the heat. Place the yolks into a medium bowl. Whisk for 2 minutes. Pour the cream over the eggs, whisking constantly. Pour the mixture back into the saucepan and place over low heat. Stir until the mixture thickens and coats the back of a spoon. Pour the mixture through a sieve into a clean bowl. Add the SomerSweet, peppermint extract, and food coloring. Stir well. Cover with plastic wrap and cool to room temperature. Refrigerate for at least 2 hours. Pour into an ice cream maker and freeze according to manufacturer's instructions.

TO ASSEMBLE

Make chocolate curls by "peeling" the chocolate bar with a vegetable peeler. Set aside. Spread the finished ice cream onto the cooled crust. Top with a layer of Perfectly Whipped Cream. Garnish with chocolate curls.

FOR THE CRUST
- 1 1/2 cups unsweetened cocoa powder
- 1/2 teaspoon baking soda
- 2 tablespoons plus 1 teaspoon SomerSweet
- 1/2 cup (1 stick) butter, chilled and cut into 1/2-inch pieces
- 1 large egg
- 1 teaspoon vanilla extract

FOR THE PEPPERMINT ICE CREAM
- 2 1/2 cups heavy cream
- 1/2 cup water
- 8 large egg yolks
- 3 tablespoons SomerSweet
- 2 tablespoons peppermint extract
- 2–3 drops green food coloring (optional)

- 1 (4.9-ounce) Somersize Milk Chocolate Baking Bar (30 squares), at room temperature
- 1 recipe Perfectly Whipped Cream (page 23)

SUGAR SUBSTITUTIONS
crust: 1/4 cup sugar
ice cream: 3/4 cup sugar
garnish: 5 ounces dark or milk chocolate

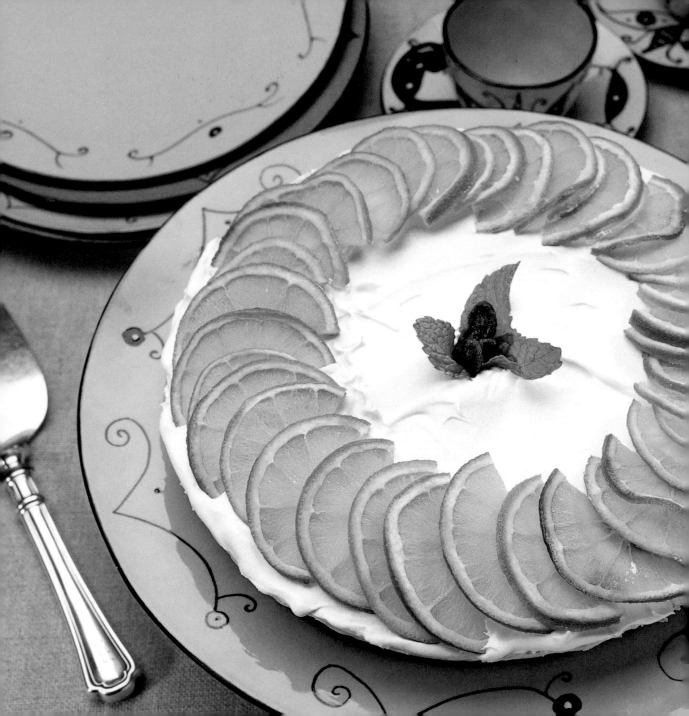

LEMON CREAM PIE WITH WHITE CHOCOLATE CRUST

ALMOST LEVEL ONE   **Makes 8 servings**

My two all-time favorite dessert flavors are white chocolate and lemon. Now they are combined in this luscious lemon pie . . . and it's so pretty.

TO MAKE CRUST

Heat the cream in a heavy saucepan until it just begins to boil. Remove from heat and stir in the chocolate until the mixture is smooth and chocolate has thoroughly melted. Stir in the lemon extract. Spread the mixture evenly in the bottom of a 9-inch glass pie pan. Refrigerate until crust has set.

TO MAKE FILLING

Beat the cream cheese and SomerSweet together until smooth. Beat in the lemon juice, zest, and food coloring. Set aside. Place the cream into a bowl and beat with an electric mixer until stiff peaks form. Fold the whipped cream into the cream cheese mixture.

Spoon the filling into the chilled chocolate crust. Cover with plastic wrap and refrigerate for at least 1 hour before serving. Garnish pie with SomerSweet Lemon Slices.

FOR THE CRUST
1/2 cup heavy cream
1 (4.9-ounce) SomerSweet
   White Chocolate Baking Bar
   (30 squares), chopped
1/2 teaspoon pure lemon
   extract

FOR THE FILLING
1 (8-ounce) package cream
   cheese, softened
1 tablespoon plus 2 teaspoons
   SomerSweet
Fresh juice and zest from
   2 lemons
1–2 drops yellow food
   coloring (optional)
1 cup heavy cream

SomerSweet Lemon Slices
   (page 69), for garnish

SUGAR SUBSTITUTIONS
crust: 5 ounces white chocolate
filling: 1/4 cup sugar

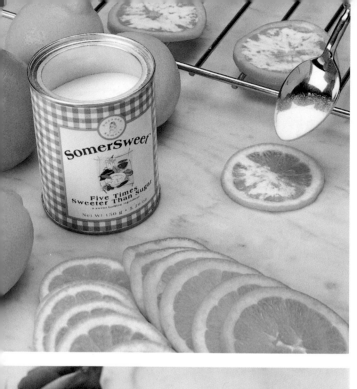
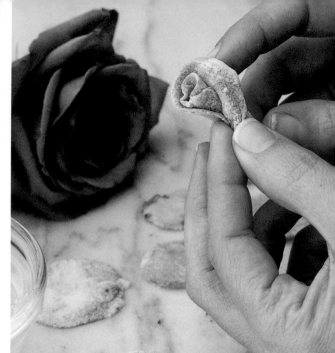
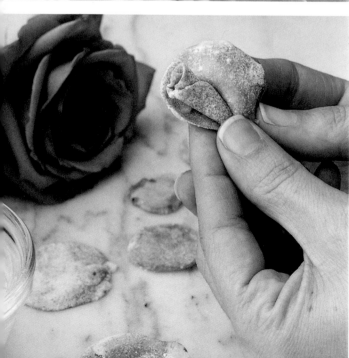
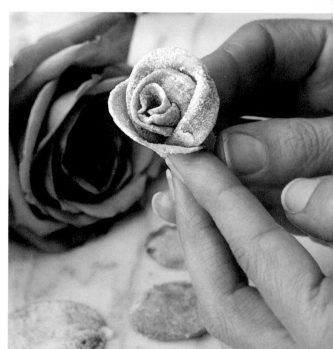

SOMERSWEET LEMON AND ORANGE SLICES
FRUIT—LEVEL ONE

Makes 8 garnishes

1 very firm lemon or orange
2 tablespoons SomerSweet

SUGAR SUBSTITUTIONS
1/2 cup sugar

I love to decorate desserts with sugared flowers or fruit—but who wants all that sugar! These lemon and orange slices are "sugared" with SomerSweet. Even better!

Preheat oven to 200°. Spray a metal rack with nonstick cooking spray, and set on top of a baking sheet.

Cut the lemon into 1/8-inch-thick slices. Blot dry on paper towels. Sprinkle with half the SomerSweet. Turn and sprinkle other sides with remaining SomerSweet. Put lemon slices onto prepared rack and place in oven for 40 to 45 minutes, or until nearly dry to the touch and just beginning to brown. If lemons brown too fast, or if they are not completely dry, turn oven off and leave lemons inside for a few hours more, or overnight. Store in an airtight container for up to 2 weeks.

SOMERSWEET ROSE PETALS
LEVEL ONE

Makes about 30

1 egg white*
2 or 3 organic roses, the
    smaller the better
2 tablespoons SomerSweet

SUGAR SUBSTITUTIONS
1/2 cup sugar

These make beautiful garnishes for nearly any dessert. After the rose petals are dry you can roll a couple together, as pictured, for a miniature flower to decorate more formal desserts.

Beat the egg white for 1 to 2 minutes in a small bowl and set aside.

Remove the petals from the roses, discarding any blemished petals. Dip each rose petal into egg white. Wipe off excess with fingers. Holding the petal over a small bowl, sprinkle with SomerSweet to coat both sides. Place petal on a fine metal rack or screen, or on a piece of waxed paper. Repeat with remaining petals. Check the petals after 20 minutes to see if there are any damp spots. If so, dip the damp spot into bowl of excess SomerSweet. Let petals sit in a warm, dry place for at least 4 hours or overnight.

To make a rosebud, take 1 SomerSweet petal and roll it, as pictured. Wrap another petal around the first, keeping the base of the petals tight and letting the tops flare out, like a flower. Continue adding petals, as desired, to create a small bud or a larger flower.

* To make the rose petals
  edible, use 2 tablespoons
  pasteurized egg white.

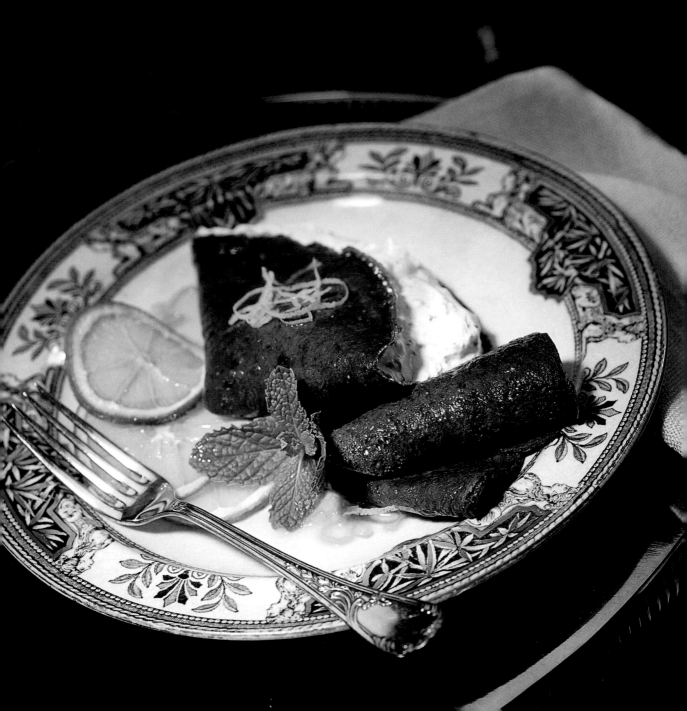

CHOCOLATE CREPES WITH MASCARPONE FILLING

ALMOST LEVEL ONE   **Makes 8 servings**

My mother-in-law, Margaret, first introduced me to Egg Crepes. They have since become a Somersize staple! Here I've turned them into Chocolate Crepes with a sweet, creamy filling and a tart orange sauce.

TO MAKE CREPES

Beat together the eggs, cocoa powder, SomerSweet, and vanilla. Set batter aside.

Heat a nonstick skillet over medium. Add ½ tablespoon butter to the pan. Pour ¼ cup of the batter into the hot skillet. Swirl the batter to evenly coat the bottom of the pan. Cook for 2 minutes. Carefully flip the crepe over and cook for 2 minutes more. Repeat with the remaining butter and batter. Stack the crepes between waxed paper and allow the crepes to cool before filling.

TO MAKE FILLING

Mix the mascarpone, SomerSweet, and grated chocolate. Spread each crepe with some filling. Fold or roll up and keep warm.

TO MAKE ORANGE SAUCE

Melt the butter, then whisk in the orange juice and SomerSweet. Heat for 2 to 3 minutes, then pour over the warm filled crepes. Garnish with fresh orange and lemon zests.

FOR THE CREPES

8 large eggs

3 tablespoons unsweetened cocoa powder

1 tablespoon plus 1 teaspoon SomerSweet

½ teaspoon vanilla extract

4 tablespoons (½ stick) butter

FOR THE FILLING

16 ounces mascarpone or cream cheese, softened

1 tablespoon plus 2 teaspoons SomerSweet

1.2 ounces or ¼ SomerSweet Milk Chocolate Baking Bar (7.5 squares), grated

FOR THE ORANGE SAUCE

½ cup (1 stick) butter

½ cup orange juice

1 teaspoon SomerSweet

Strips of orange zest and lemon zest

SUGAR SUBSTITUTIONS
crepes: 3 tablespoons sugar
crepe filling: ¼ cup sugar
3 ounces milk chocolate

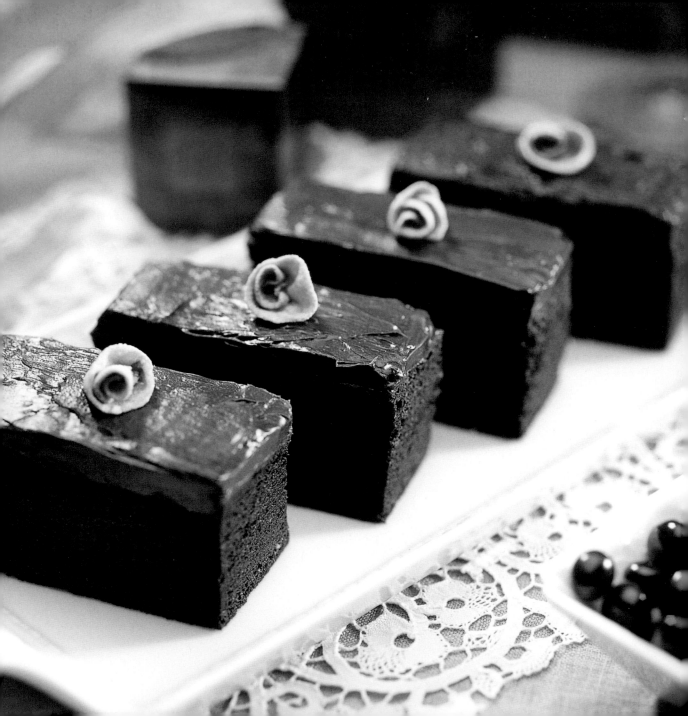

CHOCOLATE DECADENT BROWNIES WITH CHOCOLATE TRUFFLE FROSTING

ALMOST LEVEL ONE   **Makes 36 brownies**

What could be more comforting than chocolate brownies with frosting? How about chocolate brownies without the guilt! These rich, sinful treats will make you smile. They will keep for up to a week if refrigerated. Let them come to room temperature before eating for the best flavor.

Preheat oven to 400°. Line an 8-inch square baking pan with foil. Allow the foil to overhang by a few inches. Butter the foil and set pan aside.

Melt the chocolates and butter together in a double boiler over gently simmering water. Stir until chocolate is smooth. Remove from heat and allow the mixture to cool slightly.

Meanwhile, beat the eggs until pale and tripled in volume, 8 to 10 minutes (very important). Add the SomerSweet and beat for another minute. Mix one third of the egg mixture into the chocolate mixture. Carefully fold the rest of the egg mixture into the chocolate mixture. Pour into prepared pan. Pour caramel or fudge sauce on top of brownie batter and swirl in with a butter knife.

Bake for 30 minutes. The batter will not appear to be completely set. Cool completely before refrigerating. Refrigerate for at least 1 hour.

Lift the brownies out of the pan using foil as handles. Carefully peel away foil. Frost the surface of the brownies with Chocolate Truffle Frosting. Cut into 36 squares. Serve at room temperature.

2 (4.9-ounce) SomerSweet Dark Chocolate Baking Bars (60 squares), chopped

3 ounces unsweetened baking chocolate, chopped

12 tablespoons (1 1/2 sticks) unsalted butter

5 large eggs at room temperature

1 tablespoon SomerSweet

1/2 cup Somersize Caramel or Triple Fudge Sauce, warmed

1 recipe Chocolate Truffle Frosting (page 45)

SUGAR SUBSTITUTIONS
3 tablespoons sugar
10 ounces dark chocolate

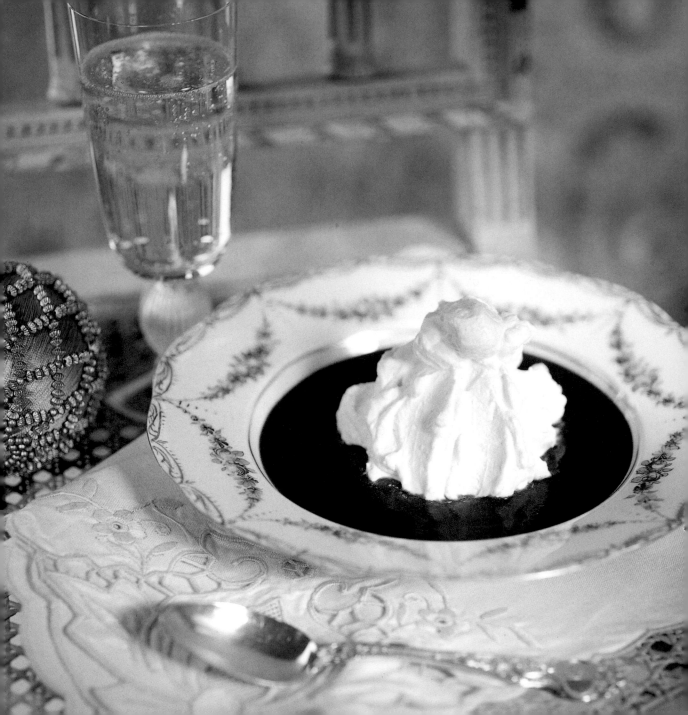

WHITE CHOCOLATE MOUSSE

ALMOST LEVEL ONE   Makes 4 servings

I have always loved chocolate mousse. Now that we have SomerSweet White Chocolate, why not White Chocolate Mousse? Yum! This is my version of a "floating island" (and it's sitting in one of my favorite china bowls).

Grate one third (10 squares) of the white chocolate and set aside. Melt the remaining two thirds (20 squares) in a double boiler or microwave. Stir until smooth. Set aside to cool slightly.

Beat the cream with an electric mixer until it begins to thicken. Add the vanilla and SomerSweet, continuing to beat until cream holds stiff peaks. Fold in the melted chocolate, then the grated chocolate. Pipe or dollop the mousse into an "island" shape on a baking sheet. Place in freezer for 15 to 20 minutes.

Place a few spoonfuls of raspberry coulis into each serving bowl. Place white chocolate mousse on each coulis and serve. (The mousse can also be simply spooned into dessert cups and chilled for at least 1 hour before serving.)

1 (4.9-ounce) SomerSweet White Chocolate Baking Bar (30 squares)
2 cups heavy cream
1 teaspoon vanilla extract
2 teaspoons SomerSweet
1 recipe Raspberry Coulis (see below)

SUGAR SUBSTITUTIONS
5 ounces white chocolate
1/2 cup sugar

RASPBERRY COULIS
FRUITS—LEVEL ONE   Makes 1 cup

Raspberry and chocolate have enjoyed a long romance as a dazzling pair. Puddle this sauce under your favorite cake, spoon it over custard, or drizzle it over ice cream.

Place all the ingredients, except the water, into a food processor and pulse until pureed. Push puree through a fine-mesh sieve to remove seeds. Adjust to the desired consistency by stirring in 1 to 2 tablespoons of water.

2 (6-ounce) baskets fresh raspberries, or 1 (12-ounce) package frozen raspberries, thawed
1 tablespoon SomerSweet
1 tablespoon lemon juice
1–2 tablespoons water, to adjust consistency

SUGAR SUBSTITUTIONS
3 tablespoons sugar

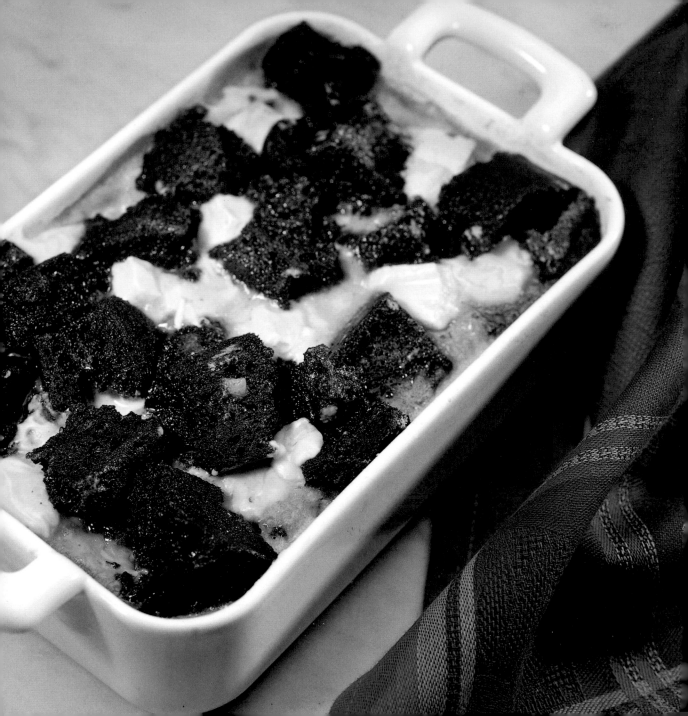

CHOCOLATE BREAD PUDDING

ALMOST LEVEL ONE   Makes 6 servings

Comfort food. Bread pudding fans will swoon over this recipe. It's chocolate bread with white chocolate chunks that ooze and melt in the custard. Oh my! During the holidays try brandy or rum extract
instead of vanilla. For shortcuts, check out my Somersize Chocolate Brownie Mix and Vanilla Pudding
Mix. Yum.

Preheat oven to 375°. Butter a 4×8-inch loaf pan and set aside.

TO MAKE CAKE

Melt the chocolates and butter together in a double boiler over gently simmering water. Stir until smooth. Remove from the heat and allow the mixture
to cool slightly. Meanwhile, beat the eggs until pale and tripled in volume, 8
to 10 minutes (very important). Add SomerSweet and beat for another
minute. Mix one third of the egg mixture into the chocolate mixture. Carefully fold the rest of the egg mixture into the chocolate mixture. Pour into
prepared pan. Bake for 30 to 35 minutes. Let cool at room temperature before
cutting into 1-inch cubes.

TO MAKE CUSTARD

Butter an 8-inch square baking dish or four 6-ounce ramekins or custard cups.
Set aside. In a mixing bowl, combine the cream, SomerSweet, eggs, vanilla,
and salt. Mix until smooth.

TO ASSEMBLE

Lower the oven temperature to 325°. Place cake pieces and white chocolate
chunks into a baking dish. Pour custard over. Let cake sit for 15 minutes to
absorb liquid. Dot surface of pudding with butter pieces. Bake for 30 to
40 minutes, or until custard has set.

FOR THE CAKE

1 (4.9-ounce) SomerSweet
   Dark Chocolate Baking Bar
   (30 squares), chopped
1½ ounces unsweetened
   baking chocolate, chopped
6 tablespoons (¾ stick)
   unsalted butter
3 large eggs at room
   temperature
2 teaspoons SomerSweet

FOR THE CUSTARD

2 cups heavy cream
3 tablespoons SomerSweet
3 large eggs
1½ teaspoons vanilla extract
⅛ teaspoon salt

TO ASSEMBLE

2.5 ounces or ½ SomerSweet
   White Chocolate Baking Bar
   (15 squares), chopped into
   ½-inch pieces
1½ tablespoons unsalted
   butter, cut into ¼-inch
   pieces

SUGAR SUBSTITUTIONS
cake: 3 tablespoons sugar
      5 ounces dark chocolate
custard: ¾ cup sugar
      3 ounces white chocolate

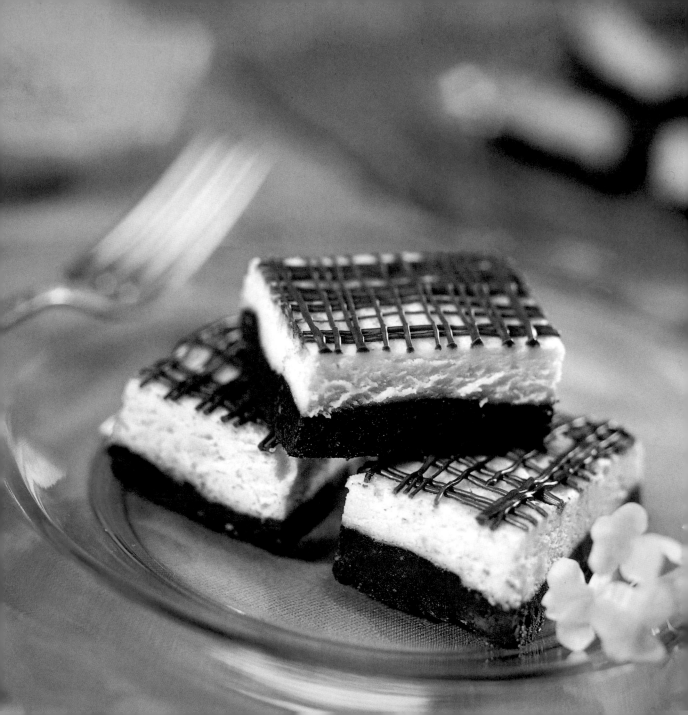

TRIPLE CHOCOLATE CREAM CHEESE BARS

ALMOST LEVEL ONE   **Makes 16 servings**

These tea bars are sweet, beautiful, and easy to make. Delicious!

TO MAKE BASE

Preheat oven to 350°. Butter an 8-inch square baking pan and set aside.

Melt the butter in a small saucepan. Add the chocolate, stirring until chocolate is melted and smooth. Remove the pan from the heat. Add the cocoa powder, SomerSweet, egg, and vanilla. Whisk until smooth. Spread the batter into the prepared pan. Bake for 15 minutes. Remove the pan from the oven and allow to cool before filling.

TO MAKE FILLING

Beat the cream cheese until light and fluffy, about 5 minutes. Add the heavy cream, SomerSweet, egg, egg yolk, vanilla, and sour cream. Beat until smooth. Pour the filling over the base. Sprinkle white chocolate over the filling and carefully stir in. Bake for 25 to 35 minutes, or until center is set. Cool completely. Cover and refrigerate for at least 2 hours or overnight.

Melt the dark or milk chocolate in the microwave, stirring every 30 seconds, until chocolate is melted and smooth. Drizzle over cooled tea bars. Cut into 16 squares.

FOR THE BASE
4 tablespoons ($^1/_2$ stick) unsalted butter
2.5 ounces or $^1/_2$ SomerSweet Dark Chocolate Baking Bar (15 squares), chopped
$^1/_3$ cup unsweetened cocoa powder
1 tablespoon SomerSweet
1 large egg
$^1/_2$ teaspoon vanilla extract

FOR THE FILLING
1 (8-ounce) package cream cheese, softened
$^1/_3$ cup heavy cream
1 tablespoon SomerSweet
1 large egg
1 large egg yolk
$^1/_2$ teaspoon vanilla extract
$^1/_4$ cup sour cream
1.8 ounces or $^1/_3$ SomerSweet White Chocolate Baking Bar (10 squares), chopped into $^1/_4$-inch pieces
2.5 ounces or $^1/_2$ SomerSweet Dark or Milk Chocolate Baking Bar (15 squares), chopped

SUGAR SUBSTITUTIONS
base: $^1/_4$ cup sugar
        3 ounces dark chocolate
filling: 2 tablespoons sugar
        3 ounces white chocolate
topping: 3 ounces milk chocolate

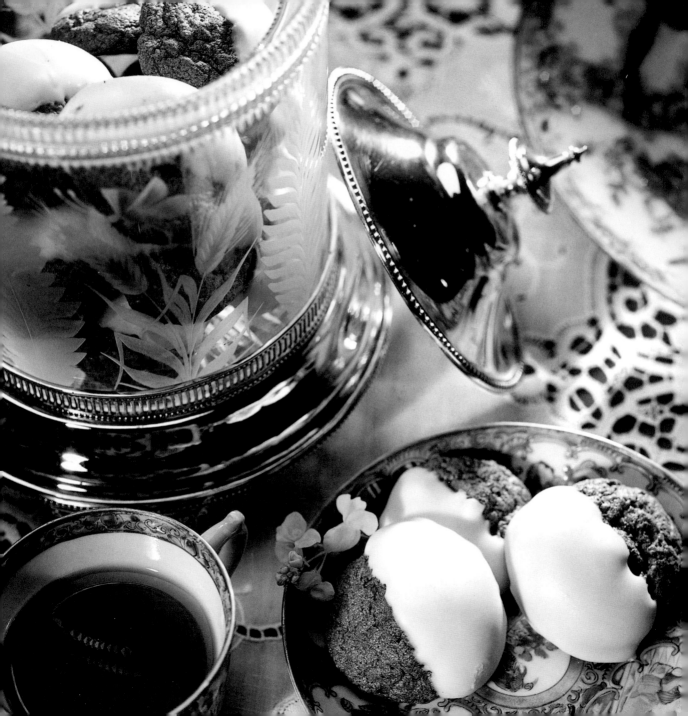

CHOCOLATE-DIPPED COCOA MERINGUE COOKIES

ALMOST LEVEL ONE   **Makes 18 cookies**

Ever since I debuted SomerSweet, I have been trying to create meringue cookies. After many failed attempts I finally figured it out! The addition of cocoa powder was the key. These light, airy cookies are perfect for afternoon tea.

Preheat oven to 250°. Line a baking sheet with parchment paper or nonstick aluminum foil and set aside.

Beat the egg whites and cream of tartar with an electric mixer until soft peaks form. Gradually add the SomerSweet while continuing to beat. Beat until the egg whites hold stiff peaks. Sift the cocoa powder onto the egg whites a little at a time. Fold in gently with a rubber scraper. Carefully fold in the grated milk chocolate. Drop the batter by the spoonful onto the prepared baking sheet. Bake for 1 hour. Turn oven off. Leave the cookies in the oven with the door closed for an additional hour. Allow cookies to cool to room temperature. Peel cookies off parchment paper.

Heat the white chocolate in a double boiler over gently simmering water, stirring until smooth. Dip cookies halfway into white chocolate. Set on a cooling rack to dry before storing at room temperature in an airtight container.

5 egg whites at room
   temperature
1/4 teaspoon cream of tartar
2 tablespoons SomerSweet
3 tablespoons unsweetened
   cocoa powder
2.5 ounces or 1/2 SomerSweet
   Milk Chocolate Baking Bar
   (15 squares), grated
1 (4.9-ounce) SomerSweet
   White Chocolate Baking Bar
   (30 squares), chopped

SUGAR SUBSTITUTIONS
1 cup sugar
3 ounces milk or dark chocolate
5 ounces white chocolate

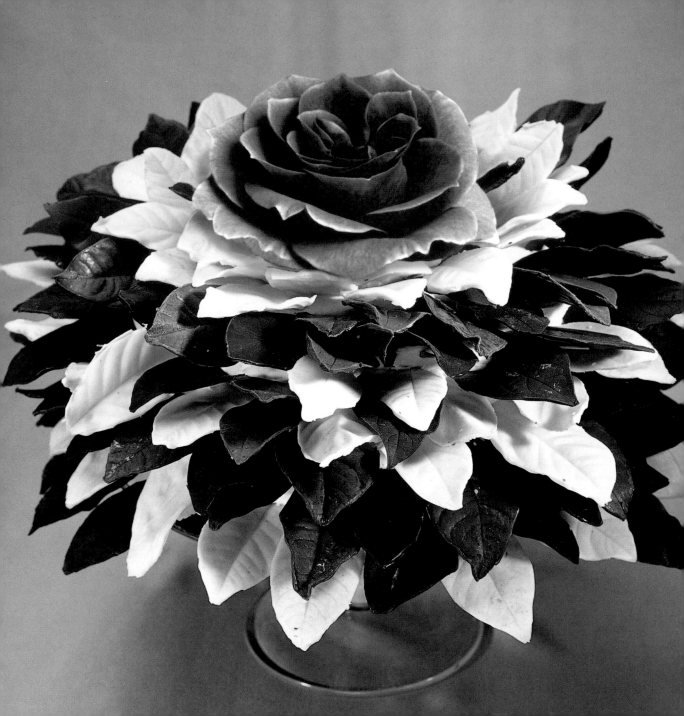

TRIPLE CHOCOLATE MOCHA MERINGUE PETAL CAKE

PRO/FATS—ALMOST LEVEL ONE   Makes 6–8 servings

This cake is a wow! The idea for this cake came to me in a dream. The next day I picked a bunch of ficus leaves, brushed them with different chocolates, and then the fun began. This is a creative experience and it is fun to spend an afternoon making it. This spectacular cake will impress the most seasoned pastry chef! Use the leaves any way you'd like to create your own fabulous design.

Preheat oven to 250°. Line the bottom of a nonstick 9-inch springform pan with waxed or parchment paper.

Place the egg whites into the clean, dry bowl of an electric mixer. (If bowl and beaters are not completely clean, egg whites will deflate. To make sure they are clean, rub with lemon juice or vinegar after washing. Rinse and dry well.) Beat on medium speed until frothy. Add the SomerSweet and beat until soft peaks form.

In a separate bowl, mix the vanilla and coffee granules. With the mixer running, gradually add the vanilla mixture to the egg whites. Continue beating until the mixture holds stiff peaks. Spoon the meringue into the prepared pan. Bake in the center of the oven for 1 hour. Remove the cake from the oven and allow to cool for 5 minutes.

Carefully run a thin-bladed knife or spatula around the edge of the cake to loosen it. Undo the spring and remove the rim of the pan. Run a spatula underneath the cake to loosen it before removing from the bottom of the pan. Remove the waxed paper from the bottom of the cake. Allow to cool completely before decorating.

Pour the warm fudge sauce on top of the cake. The sauce will make a puddle in the center of the cake. Beat the cream with the electric mixer until it forms stiff peaks. Fold the warm caramel sauce into the whipped cream. Smooth the caramel cream over the top and sides of the cake. Or generously dollop the caramel cream onto slices of cake before serving. Decorate with Chocolate Leaves. Support underside of leaves with toothpicks, as needed.

9 large egg whites at room temperature
1/3 cup SomerSweet
2 teaspoons vanilla extract
2 tablespoons instant decaf coffee granules
1/2 cup Somersize Triple Hot Fudge Sauce, slightly warmed
2 cups whipping cream
1/2 cup Somersize Caramel Sauce, slightly warmed
Chocolate Leaves (page 85; see Note below)

SUGAR SUBSTITUTIONS
2 cups sugar

NOTE: You can make the Chocolate Leaves in advance and freeze them until ready to use.

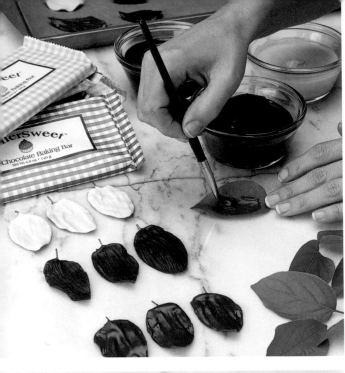
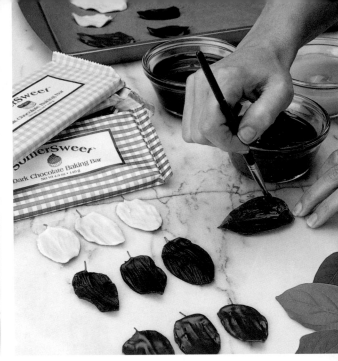
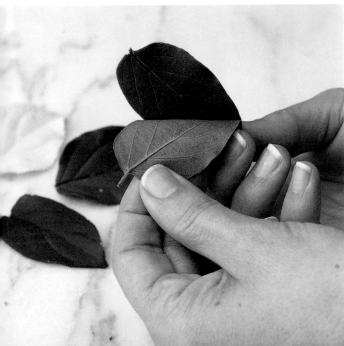
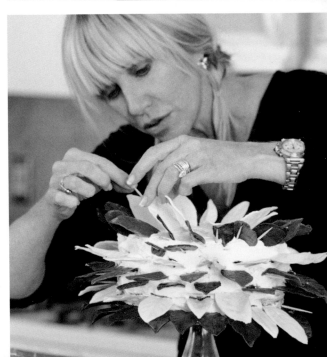

CHOCOLATE LEAVES
ALMOST LEVEL ONE   **Makes about 2 dozen leaves**

I like to have these beautiful leaves on hand in my freezer to decorate cakes when unexpected guests drop by. For best results, make sure you use stiff, nonpoisonous leaves (rose leaves, lemon or lime leaves, camellia or gardenia leaves) with well-defined veins.

Line a baking sheet with waxed paper or foil and set aside. Melt chocolate in a double boiler over gently simmering water, stirring until smooth.

Using a pastry brush, carefully coat the underside of the leaf with melted chocolate. Wipe away any chocolate overflow from the edges. Place the leaf, chocolate side up, on the prepared baking sheet. Repeat with remaining leaves. Refrigerate the leaves until the chocolate is cold and set, about 10 minutes.

Carefully peel the leaves off the chocolate and return the chocolate leaves to the baking sheet. Freeze or refrigerate until ready to use.

1 (4.9-ounce) SomerSweet White, Milk, or Dark Chocolate Baking Bar (30 squares), finely chopped

24 fresh stiff leaves, wiped clean with moist paper towels and patted dry

SUGAR SUBSTITUTIONS
5 ounces milk, dark, or white chocolate

Index

About the Author

SUZANNE SOMERS is the author of twelve books, including the *New York Times* bestsellers *Keeping Secrets; Eat Great, Lose Weight; Get Skinny on Fabulous Food; Eat, Cheat, and Melt the Fat Away; Suzanne Somers' Fast and Easy;* and *The Sexy Years.* The former star of the hit television programs *Three's Company* and *Step by Step,* Suzanne is one of the most respected and trusted brand names in the world, representing cosmetics and skincare products, apparel, jewelry, a computerized facial fitness system, fitness products, and a dessert line called SomerSweet. She received an Honorary Doctorate of Humane Letters from National University and is a highly sought-after commencement speaker.